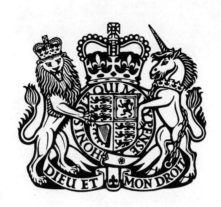

The Law Commission
Consultation Paper No 137

COMMON AND PUBLIC LAW

LIABILITY FOR PSYCHIATRIC ILLNESS

A CONSULTATION PAPER

HMSO

Printed in the United Kingdom for HMSO
Dd297932 3/95 C18 G559 10170

THE LAW COMMISSION

LIABILITY FOR PSYCHIATRIC ILLNESS

CONTENTS

[Handwritten annotation next to item (2): "Page v. Smith"; "a psychiatric illness" is boxed]

iii

personal

PART I
INTRODUCTION

1.1 This is the third consultation paper in our "examination of the principles governing and the effectiveness of the present remedy of damages for monetary and non-monetary loss, with particular regard to personal injury litigation".[1] This paper differs from those so far published under Item 11 of our Fifth Programme of Law Reform in focusing on liability rather than the assessment of damages.[2] It became clear during our work on the assessment of damages for non-pecuniary loss[3] that there was widespread concern over this area of personal injury litigation, especially following the decision of the House of Lords in the leading case of *Alcock v Chief Constable of South Yorkshire Police*.[4] We therefore concluded that a review of damages "with particular regard to personal injury litigation" should address the problem of negligently inflicted psychiatric illness.

1.2 Traditionally the term "nervous shock" has been used to describe the harm in question. But more recently that term has been strongly criticised as "crude",[5] "quaint",[6] and as a "misleading and inaccurate expression".[7] It probably entered judicial vocabulary as a result of medical experts having used the expression when giving evidence and was closely intertwined with the concept of shock in medical terms, for example "shell shock", the precursor to "post-traumatic stress disorder".[8] Arguably it remains a convenient label in indicating that, to be compensatable, a

---

[1] Item 11 of our Fifth Programme of Law Reform (1991) Law Com No 200. We explain in the description of Item 11 that we are looking only at the remedy of damages as applicable within the traditional common law system and that we shall not be considering alternative forms of compensation outside that system.

[2] Other published papers are the consultation papers: Structured Settlements and Interim and Provisional Damages (1992) Consultation Paper No 125, and Aggravated, Exemplary and Restitutionary Damages (1993) Consultation Paper No 132, and the Reports: Structured Settlements and Interim and Provisional Damages (1994) Law Com No 224, and Personal Injury Compensation: How Much is Enough? (1994) Law Com No 225.

[3] We hope to publish a consultation paper on damages for non-pecuniary loss in personal injury cases in the Summer of 1995.

[4] [1992] 1 AC 310.

[5] *Jaensch v Coffey* (1984) 155 CLR 549, 552, *per* Gibbs CJ.

[6] *McLoughlin v O'Brian* [1983] 1 AC 410, 432, *per* Lord Bridge.

[7] *Attia v British Gas Plc* [1988] QB 304, 317, *per* Bingham LJ (who preferred the term "psychiatric damage"). See also *Jaensch v Coffey* (1984) 155 CLR 549, 560, *per* Brennan J. In his foreword to N J Mullany and P R Handford, *Tort Liability for Psychiatric Damage* (1993) p vii, Sir Thomas Bingham MR criticised the label "nervous shock" because it is "not only misleading and inaccurate but, with its echoes of frail Victorian heroines, tends to disguise the very serious damage which is, in many cases, under discussion." In *Page v Smith* [1994] 4 All ER 522, 549 Hoffmann LJ said that the term "nervous shock" had "gone out of fashion".

[8] Paras 3.5-3.9 below. C Pugh and M Trimble, "Psychiatric Injury after Hillsborough" (1993) 163 British Journal of Psychiatry 425.

psychiatric illness must usually be the result of shock or trauma.[9] However, psychiatric illness is sometimes compensatable even where not shock-induced; and, even where it is insisted that the psychiatric illness be shock-induced, one of the very questions we wish to address is whether that should continue to be a requirement. We have therefore thought it preferable to use the wider, and less controversial, phrase "psychiatric illness" rather than "nervous shock".

1.3 We are not concerned in this paper with psychiatric illness consequent on physical injury to the plaintiff. Compensation for such psychiatric illness (for example, depression following loss of a limb[10]) is as recoverable as for any other personal injury and there are no special restrictions on liability.[11] Nor are we concerned with the situation where a shock to the plaintiff has caused a physical injury that is distinct from any psychiatric illness and the plaintiff claims damages for the distinct physical injury, for example, where the shock of witnessing an horrific event is such that the plaintiff suffers a stroke.[12] Here again damages are as recoverable for the physical injury as for any other personal injury.[13]

1.4 Also outside the scope of this paper is psychiatric illness caused by an intentional tort. In *Wilkinson v Downton*[14] the defendant deliberately and falsely told the plaintiff, as a practical joke, that her husband had been injured in a road accident. The plaintiff suffered a severe shock and was seriously ill for some time. She was able to recover in tort for the "physical harm" resulting from the defendant's wilful act. The physical harm in this case was a psychiatric illness.[15] An action based on the *Wilkinson* case evades the restrictions on a negligence action for psychiatric illness. Indeed *Wilkinson* is probably authority for the general proposition that

---

[9] *Alcock v Chief Constable of South Yorkshire Police* [1992] 1 AC 310, 351, *per* Parker LJ. See also *Brice v Brown* [1984] 1 All ER 997, 1006 and J Swanton, "Issues in Tort Liability for Nervous Shock" (1992) 66 ALJ 495. The point has also been made that the phrase "nervous shock" allows the judge the freedom of manoeuvre which is a valuable part of his or her function: C Gearty, " Tort - Nervous Shock - 'Eggshell Skull' Rules, O.K.?" [1984] CLJ 238, 240.

[10] Another example is "compensation neurosis" consequent on physical injury: see eg, *James v Woodall Duckham Construction Co Ltd* [1969] 1 WLR 903.

[11] *Jaensch v Coffey* (1984) 155 CLR 549, 593, *per* Deane J; M Jones, *Textbook on Torts* (4th ed 1993) p 101.

[12] As in, eg, *Galt v British Railways Board* (1983) 133 NLJ 870 (heart attack).

[13] N J Mullany and P R Handford, *Tort Liability for Psychiatric Damage* (1993) p 18; *Winfield and Jolowicz on Tort* (14th ed 1994) p 119, n 16. Cf *Winfield and Jolowicz on Tort* (13th ed 1989) p 107; *Page v Smith* [1994] 4 All ER 522, 549, *per* Hoffmann LJ.

[14] [1897] 2 QB 57. See generally *Winfield and Jolowicz on Tort* (14th ed 1994) pp 74-75; B S Markesinis & S F Deakin, *Tort Law* (3rd ed 1994) pp 367-368; and N J Mullany and P R Handford, *Tort Liability for Psychiatric Damage* (1993) ch 14.

[15] As it was in *Janvier v Sweeney* [1919] 2 KB 316 in which *Wilkinson v Downton* was followed. Mullany and Handford point out that there have been only a few *Wilkinson v Downton* cases in Commonwealth countries but a vast number in the United States: *Tort Liability for Psychiatric Damage* (1993) p 307.

intentional or reckless conduct aimed at the plaintiff and resulting in personal injury can found an action in tort, even though the "indirectness" of the harm means that there is no action for trespass to the person.[16] Whatever the precise scope of *Wilkinson* - and it seems eminently suited to further *judicial* refinement - it is axiomatic that damages for psychiatric illness are, for this form of liability, as recoverable as for any other personal injury.

1.5   Our concern therefore is almost exclusively with the tort of negligence. In past cases it is in relation to the tort of negligence that psychiatric illness has been regarded as raising problems. Nevertheless, despite the lack of case law outside the realm of negligence, it seems in principle that the special restrictions developed for the recovery of psychiatric illness for negligence ought to extend to the recovery of damages for psychiatric illness for closely related torts, for example, liability under the Occupiers' Liability Acts 1957 and 1984; and possibly even to torts of strict liability, for example *Rylands v Fletcher* liability or liability under the Animals Act 1971 or under the Consumer Protection Act 1987.[17] This paper is therefore concerned with the recovery of damages for psychiatric illness in the tort of negligence and in respect of any other tort (or, conceivably, a non-tortious cause of action, such as breach of confidence) for which special restrictions on liability for psychiatric illness, analogous to those in negligence, are applicable. We should add that, on our understanding of the present law, while contractual damages for mere mental distress are indisputably only recoverable in limited circumstances,[18] no special restrictions are placed on the recovery of contractual damages for psychiatric illness.[19] In other words, in actions for breach of contract psychiatric illness appears

[16]   The case has recently been controversially relied on as authority for the grant of an injunction in cases of harassment or molestation by means such as threatening telephone calls, where injury to the health of the victim is likely to result (*Khorasandjian v Bush* [1993] QB 727).

[17]   Presumably damages for psychiatric illness are recoverable without special restrictions for the tort of private nuisance (eg, psychiatric illness brought on by noise or by the spread of fire or by hill-creep) because, in contrast to the tort of negligence, damages for mental distress (loss of enjoyment of the use of one's land) are recoverable. See, eg, *Pelmothe v Phillips* (1899) 20 LR (NSW) 58. On the recovery of damages for personal injury generally in private nuisance and under *Rylands v Fletcher*, see *Winfield and Jolowicz on Tort* (14th ed 1994) pp 419-420, 450-451. Damages for psychiatric illness are presumably recoverable for the tort of defamation as, again, damages for mental distress are recoverable. Note that as, under s 1(9) of the Occupiers' Liability Act 1984, s 11 of the Animals Act 1971 and s 45(1) of the Consumer Protection Act 1987, "damage" or "injury" is defined to mean, or include, "any impairment of physical or mental condition" it is not clear that special common law restrictions can be imposed in the context of claims brought under those statutes.

[18]   Ie where the predominant object of the contract was to obtain mental satisfaction or where the mental distress is directly consequent on physical inconvenience: see, eg, *Jarvis v Swans Tours Ltd* [1973] QB 233; *Bliss v South East Thames Regional Health Authority* [1985] IRLR 308, 316; *Hayes v James & Charles Dodd* [1990] 2 All ER 815; *Watts v Morrow* [1991] 1 WLR 1421.

[19]   See, eg, *Cook v Swinfen* [1967] 1 WLR 457; *Malyon v Lawrance, Messer & Co* [1968] 2 Lloyd's Rep 539. See *McGregor on Damages* (15th ed 1988) paras 94-95; G H Treitel, *The Law of Contract* (8th ed 1991) p 879; *Jackson & Powell on Professional Negligence* (3rd ed

to be treated like any other personal injury. If that is correct the most obvious justification for it is that, with contractual claims, there is no fear of opening the floodgates of litigation in the major sense of there being an indeterminate number of claims from a single breach.[20]

1.6 **We would welcome the views of consultees as to the torts (or, conceivably, non-tortious causes of action) in respect of which liability for psychiatric illness attracts special restrictions (ie restrictions that are not applied to liability for physical injury). In particular we would be pleased to hear from practitioners who have encountered such special restrictions in respect of claims for psychiatric illness not based on the tort of negligence. We would also be grateful for views as to whether we are correct in our understanding that, in actions for breach of contract, no special restrictions are placed on the recovery of damages for psychiatric illness and whether, if that is so, consultees consider, as we do, that that is a justified approach for the law to take.**

1.7 Recently public interest in negligently caused psychiatric illness and the circumstances in which it may give rise to a claim for damages has been awakened by a number of high-profile cases,[21] and especially by the disaster at the Hillsborough football stadium in which 95 spectators were killed and over 400 injured by crushing caused when spectators were permitted to continue to enter a terrace that was already full. In test cases culminating in the decision of the House of Lords in *Alcock v Chief Constable of South Yorkshire Police*[22] various relatives and friends of people at the match claimed damages for psychiatric illness. All but one were ultimately unsuccessful.

1.8 For some 90 years it has been recognised by the courts that negligently caused psychiatric illness (standing alone) can give rise to a claim for damages.[23] During this time, the relevant law has undergone radical development, albeit incrementally, with the trend being one of a gradual widening of liability. Lord Oliver in the *Alcock* case stated that he did not "regard the present state of the law as either entirely satisfactory or as logically defensible" and that "the ultimate boundaries within

---

1992) para 4-211; *Chitty on Contracts* (27th ed 1994) vol I, para 26-041.

[20] See para 4.2 below.

[21] See, eg, *Walker v Northumberland CC* (1994) 144 NLJ 1659 (para 2.49 below); and *Vernon v Bosley*, unreported, 30 January 1995 (para 2.54 n 169 below).

[22] [1992] 1 AC 310. See paras 2.18-2.19 below for an outline of the decision. Claims have also been brought by a number of police officers who were on duty at Hillsborough. Out-of-court settlements have been reached in respect of a number of those claims (see para 2.27 n 91) and others are due to be heard in late March 1995.

[23] *Dulieu v White & Sons* [1901] 2 KB 669. In the earlier case of *Victorian Railways Commissioners v Coultas* (1888) 13 App Cas 222 such liability had been denied.

which claims for damages in such cases can be entertained must ... depend in the end upon considerations of policy".[24] Sir Thomas Bingham MR has described the subject as "one of the most vexed and tantalising topics in the modern law of tort" and has pointed out that:

> "Underlying the cases has been the judges' concern that unless the limits of liability are tightly drawn the courts will be inundated with a flood of claims by plaintiffs ever more distant from the scene of the original mishap. So fine distinctions have been drawn and strict lines of demarcation established."[25]

The difficulty of drawing the policy line or cut-off point for liability for psychiatric illness has given rise in turn to calls for Parliament to consider the competing aspects of public policy and for the rights of persons who sustain negligently inflicted psychiatric illness to be enshrined in legislation.[26] Whilst others have expressed the view that legislative limits to recovery for psychiatric illness would be unduly rigid, they have nevertheless acknowledged the need for reform of this area of the law, in particular, for an expansion of liability and the removal of unnecessary hurdles to recovery.[27] In this paper we consider whether there is scope for reform of the common law and whether development should continue to be by the courts or requires legislation, as in a number of Australian jurisdictions.

1.9   We are aware from our preliminary consultations that there are strongly-held views on this topic. On the one hand, there are those who are sceptical about the award of damages for psychiatric illness. They argue that such illness can easily be faked; that, in any event, those who are suffering should be able "to pull themselves together"; and that, even if they cannot do so, there is no good reason why

---

[24]   [1992] 1 AC 310, 418.

[25]   Foreword to N J Mullany and P R Handford, *Tort Liability for Psychiatric Damage* (1993) p vii. See, similarly, his comments in *M v Newham LBC* [1994] 2 WLR 554, 573.

[26]   *Alcock v Chief Constable of South Yorkshire Police* [1992] 1 AC 310, 417, 419, *per* Lord Oliver; *McLoughlin v O'Brian* [1983] 1 AC 410, 429-431, *per* Lord Scarman; and see Stocker LJ in the Court of Appeal in *Alcock*: [1992] 1 AC 310, 376. See also K J Nasir, "Nervous Shock and *Alcock*: The Judicial Buck Stops Here" (1992) 55 MLR 705, 707, 713; A Watson, "Recovery for Nervous Shock: A Look at the Law and Some Thoughts of Reform" (1993) 12 Lit 193, 200; J Cooke, "One Step Forward, Two Steps Back? - Nervous Shock and the Hillsborough Disaster" [1991] 13(2) Liverpool LR 201, 211.

[27]   *McLoughlin v O'Brian* [1983] 1 AC 410, 431, 441-443, *per* Lord Bridge. See also N J Mullany and P R Handford, *Tort Liability for Psychiatric Damage* (1993) pp ix, 245, 311; *Salmond & Heuston on the Law of Torts* (20th ed 1992) pp 222-223; A Unger, "Undue caution in the Lords" (1991) 141 NLJ 1729, 1730; F A Trindade, "The Principles Governing the Recovery of Damages for Negligently Caused Nervous Shock" [1986] CLJ 476; C Pugh and M Trimble, "Psychiatric Injury after Hillsborough" (1993) 163 British Journal of Psychiatry 425, 428-429.

defendants and, through them, those who pay insurance premiums should pay for their inability to do so.[28] As Birkett J observed in a case in the 1940's:

> "I quite recognise that when we are in this field, it is a very difficult one for laymen to understand. When witnesses speak about a man suffering from an ... anxiety neurosis when a man is not suffering organically but has hysteria, the ordinary, sound, healthy man is apt to look upon that with a little disdain or a little suspicion and to treat it sometimes rather lightly and to say: 'Well, if you have a little courage or determination you can overcome it. If you have a little will-power to go back to work and confront the difficulty, that would overcome it'."[29]

On the other hand, medical and legal experts working in the field, who are the people who most commonly encounter those complaining of psychiatric illness, have impressed upon us how life-shattering psychiatric illness can be and how, in many instances, it can be more debilitating than physical injuries.

1.10   The rest of the paper is arranged as follows. In Part II we set out the present law. Part III contains a brief exposition of the medical background. Part IV examines the policy arguments underlying the cautious approach which has been adopted by the courts. Part V sets out the issues and options for reform. Part VI summarises the reform issues and gathers together our provisional conclusions. The law in a number of other jurisdictions is summarised in the Appendix.

1.11   We gratefully acknowledge the invaluable assistance of:- Dr Sally Lloyd-Bostock of the Centre for Socio-Legal Studies, Wolfson College, Oxford, Dr Richard Mayou and Dr Bridget Bryant of Warneford Hospital, Oxford, Dr Nigel Eastman of St George's Hospital Medical School, London, and Dr Stuart Turner of University College & Middlesex Hospital School of Medicine, London, all of whom helped us with the medical aspects of this paper; and Mr J W Davies of Brasenose College, Oxford, who commented on a draft of this paper. We would also like to thank Nicholas Mullany and Dr Peter Handford for the great help that we have derived

---

[28]   For examples of this sort of view, see the editorials "Damaging us all" and "Moral blackmail" in the *Daily Telegraph* of 1 and 3 February 1995, criticising the decision of Sedley J in *Vernon v Bosley*, unreported, 30 January 1995 (see para 2.54 n 169) and the out-of-court settlement of some of the claims by police officers who were on duty at Hillsborough (see para 2.27 n 91).

[29]   *Griffiths v R & H Green and Silley Weir Ltd* (1948) 81 Ll L Rep 378, 380 (on the facts of the case there was no real difficulty over liability, as opposed to quantum, because the plaintiff's alleged psychiatric illness was consequent on a physical injury, namely a blow to the head suffered in an accident at work).

from their meticulously researched book, *Tort Liability for Psychiatric Damage* (1993).[30]

---

[30] In addition to the book itself, we have derived assistance from the large number of reviews of it. These include: H Teff (1994) 10 PN 108; J G Fleming (1994) 2 Tort Law Review 202; P Cane (1993) 23 Univ of Western Australia LR 378; R Bagshaw (1993) 109 LQR 691; D W Robertson (1994) 57 MLR 649; T Weir [1993] CLJ 520; K Stanton (1994) Anglo-American LR 249; N Solomon (1994) 1 JPIL 169; M Lunney (1993) 1 Med LR 408; M McInnes (1993) 16 Dalhousie LJ 494; S Todd (1993) 15 NZULR 466; G H L Fridman (1994) 73 Can BR 110; B A Hocking (1994) 1 Psychiatry, Psychology and Law 59; L W Maher (1993) 19 Melbourne Univ LR 244; T Plewman (1994) 111 SALJ 213; L Skene (1994) 2 Tort LJ 96; and G Seabourne (1994) 14 Legal Studies 283. The review by M McInnes concludes with the following paragraph:

> "Finally, *Tort Liability for Psychiatric Damage* draws upon the compelling, often tragic, facts that have given rise to actions for psychiatric illness. Claims have been pursued as a result of being denied a make-up examination in a Criminal Procedure course, being attacked by a chimpanzee, learning of a sister's death through 'extra-sensory empathy', watching a relative's coffin tumble out of the back of a hearse, and witnessing a ceremonial circumcision go terribly wrong. Mullany & Handford's text is consequently not only among the best written and most informative works on the market, it is also among the most readable."

PART II
THE PRESENT LAW

INTRODUCTION

2.1 Although liability in tort for negligently inflicted psychiatric illness can be traced back to the beginning of the century,[1] it was only in 1942 in *Bourhill v Young*[2] that this development was authoritatively established as valid by a decision of the House of Lords. However, in that case Lord Macmillan said that "[I]n the case of mental shock there are elements of greater subtlety than in the case of an ordinary physical injury and these elements may give rise to debate as to the precise scope of legal liability".[3] Liability for negligently caused psychiatric illness has subsequently been considered twice by the House of Lords: in *McLoughlin v O'Brian*[4] in 1982, and in *Alcock v Chief Constable of South Yorkshire Police*[5] in 1991. It is difficult to say that those cases, and others in the lower courts, have now settled the precise scope of legal liability but a tolerably clear picture of the relevant principles has emerged.

PRINCIPLES OF LIABILITY

2.2 The problematic liability issues in this sphere have almost always been seen as going to the question whether the defendant owed the plaintiff a duty of care.[6] In contrast the legal principles applicable to the other central elements of the tort of negligence — that is, that the defendant's conduct was negligent, that it caused the plaintiff's psychiatric illness, that that illness was not too remote applying the *Wagon Mound* test,[7] and that there is no defence[8] — are relatively non-problematic, being applied in the same way to psychiatric illness as to a physical injury.[9] They need not detain us further.

> Is this true? — see David Carson?
> also, cf *Page v Smith*.
> Do 'causation' probs drive the 'policy' probs?

---

[1] *Dulieu v White & Sons* [1901] 2 KB 669.

[2] [1943] AC 92.

[3] *Ibid*, 103.

[4] [1983] 1 AC 410.

[5] [1992] 1 AC 310.

[6] An exception is *Attia v British Gas Plc* [1988] QB 304 in which, in a case concerned with psychiatric illness consequent on damage to property, the Court of Appeal found it more convenient to analyse the issues in terms of remoteness of damage. See *Winfield & Jolowicz on Tort* (14th ed 1994) pp 123-124.

[7] [1961] AC 388.

[8] Eg volenti non fit injuria, exclusion of liability, illegality.

[9] For a note of caution as regards causation, see P Cane, Book Review of N J Mullany and P R Handford, *Tort Liability for Psychiatric Damage* (1993) 23 Univ of Western Australia LR 378, 379: "There is very little discussion [in the book] of how to go about establishing a causal link between mental injury and external event - an issue which must, in practice, often be of great and crucial difficulty."

2.3 On the assumption, then, that applying normal principles the plaintiff can establish negligence, causation, that the harm is not too remote, and that there are no defences ruling out liability, the present law can be largely encapsulated in the following seven propositions:[10]

(1) The plaintiff must have suffered a recognised psychiatric illness that, at least where the plaintiff is a secondary victim, must be shock-induced.

(2) It must have been reasonably foreseeable that the plaintiff might suffer a psychiatric illness as a result of the defendant's negligence.

(3) The plaintiff can recover if the foreseeable psychiatric illness arose from a reasonable fear of immediate physical injury to himself or herself.

(4) Where the defendant has negligently injured or imperilled someone other than the plaintiff (but probably excluding the defendant himself or herself) and the plaintiff, as a result, has foreseeably suffered a shock-induced psychiatric illness, the plaintiff can recover if he or she can establish the requisite degree of proximity in terms of:

(a) the class of persons whose claims should be recognised and

(b) the closeness of the plaintiff to the accident in time and space and

(c) the means by which the shock is caused.

(5) Where the defendant has negligently damaged or imperilled property belonging to the plaintiff or a third party, and the plaintiff, as a result, has foreseeably suffered a psychiatric illness, it would appear that, in certain circumstances, the plaintiff can recover for that illness but the necessary criteria for recovery are unclear.

(6) It is unclear whether there can be liability for the negligent communication of news to the plaintiff which has foreseeably caused him or her to suffer a psychiatric illness.

(7) There are miscellaneous instances (that is, other than those covered by propositions (3) (5) and (6) above) where a primary victim probably

---

[10] As will be apparent, propositions (1) and (2) lay down pre-conditions for the application of propositions (3) to (7).

can recover for a psychiatric illness foreseeably caused by the defendant's negligence.

We shall consider each of those propositions in turn.

(1) The plaintiff must suffer a recognised psychiatric illness that, at least where the plaintiff is a secondary victim, must be shock-induced.

2.4 The plaintiff must establish that he or she is suffering from a recognised psychiatric illness.[11] Lesser mental harm, such as grief, fear, anxiety, vexation, and distress, does not suffice.[12] Damages are not recoverable for a "shock" in itself, which was no more than an immediate emotional response to a distressing experience, however sudden, severe and saddening, although such a shock can be the starting point of a psychiatric disorder.[13] In past cases the types of recognised psychiatric illness that have qualified for this cause of action have included "reactive depression",[14] "pathological grief",[15] "hysterical personality disorder",[16] and "post-traumatic stress disorder".[17] Expert medical evidence will normally be necessary to establish that the plaintiff has suffered a recognised psychiatric illness.

---

[11] *Hinz v Berry* [1970] 2 QB 40, 42, *per* Lord Denning MR; *McLoughlin v O'Brian* [1983] 1 AC 410, 418, *per* Lord Wilberforce; 431, *per* Lord Bridge.

[12] *Alcock v Chief Constable of South Yorkshire Police* [1992] 1 AC 310, 401, *per* Lord Ackner; 408-410 and 416, *per* Lord Oliver; *Hinz v Berry* [1970] 2 QB 40, 42, *per* Lord Denning MR; *McLoughlin v O'Brian* [1983] 1 AC 410, 431, *per* Lord Bridge. Fear, therefore, of whatever degree, will not be sufficient: *Hicks v Chief Constable of the South Yorkshire Police* [1992] 2 All ER 65, 69, *per* Lord Bridge; *Nicholls v Rushton, The Times* 19 June 1992 (no question of damages in negligence for severe shock and shaking up falling short of an identifiable psychiatric illness where there was no physical injury or trauma). See also, *Calveley v Chief Constable of the Merseyside Police* [1989] AC 1228, 1238 (Lord Bridge) (no claim in negligence for mere anxiety, vexation and injury to reputation); *Kerby v Redbridge Health Authority* [1994] PIQR Q1 (no damages recoverable in negligence for "dashed hopes" of plaintiff in respect of death of new-born baby owing to defendants' negligence).

[13] *Mount Isa Mines Ltd v Pusey* (1970) 125 CLR 383, 394-395, *per* Windeyer J. See, however, the controversial decision in *Whitmore v Euroways Express Coaches Ltd, The Times* 4 May 1984, where the plaintiff recovered damages for ordinary shock not amounting to a psychiatric condition which she suffered on witnessing injury to her husband: the decision is generally regarded as an aberration.

[14] *Hevican v Ruane* [1991] 3 All ER 65, 67. But see para 2.33 below.

[15] *Alcock v Chief Constable of South Yorkshire Police* [1992] 1 AC 310, 365, *per* Stocker LJ; *Tredget v Bexley HA* [1994] 5 Med LR 178 (County Ct).

[16] *Brice v Brown* [1984] 1 All ER 997, 1004.

[17] *Alcock v Chief Constable of South Yorkshire Police* [1992] 1 AC 310, 365, *per* Stocker LJ. It is this type of psychiatric illness that most commonly features in claims for damages: see para 3.5 below. In *M v Newham LBC* [1994] 2 WLR 554 Sir Thomas Bingham MR, dissenting, recognised "anxiety neurosis" as an actionable psychiatric illness, see para 2.6 below; and in *McLoughlin v O'Brian* [1983] 1 AC 410, 431, Lord Bridge also recognised that anxiety neurosis could be an actionable psychiatric illness.

2.5   Damages are in general only recoverable where the recognised psychiatric illness was shock-induced. What is required is "a sudden assault on the nervous system"[18] or "the sudden appreciation ... of a horrifying event, which violently agitates the mind".[19] The law does not in general provide recovery for psychiatric illness brought about by an accumulation of more gradual assaults upon the nervous system. A person who has had to cope with the deprivation consequent upon a bereavement,[20] a spouse who has been worn down by caring for an injured husband or wife, and a parent made distraught by the wayward conduct of a brain-damaged child are not able to claim for psychiatric illness suffered as a result.[21]

2.6   In *M v Newham London Borough Council*,[22] in which the plaintiffs, a child and her mother, allegedly suffered "anxiety neurosis" as a result of having been separated for a year on the basis of a false psychiatric report that the child was being sexually abused by the mother's boyfriend, Sir Thomas Bingham MR, dissenting, thought that the child's negligence claim should not be struck out even though the psychiatric illness was not the result of a sudden occurrence.[23] He gave three reasons for departing from the traditional view as authoritatively confirmed by Lord Ackner in *Alcock*.[24] First, that Lord Ackner had acknowledged that future

[18]   *Alcock v Chief Constable of South Yorkshire Police* [1992] 1 AC 310, 398, *per* Lord Keith.

[19]   *Alcock v Chief Constable of South Yorkshire Police* [1992] 1 AC 310, 401, *per* Lord Ackner. On the facts of *Alcock* - see paras 2.18-2.19 below - it is arguable that all the plaintiffs satisfied the requirement of having suffered shock-induced psychiatric illness; but cf Lord Oliver's speech, at pp 417-418, which can be read as ruling out the claims because the shock was gradual rather than sudden.

[20]   *Alcock v Chief Constable of South Yorkshire Police* [1992] 1 AC 310, 400, *per* Lord Ackner. See also *Taylorson v Shieldness Produce Ltd* [1994] PIQR P329 (para 2.31 n 105 below); and *Calascione v Dixon*, 30 July 1993 (CA), *Kemp and Kemp* vol 2, para C4-151, in which damages for pathological grief reaction (as opposed to post-traumatic stress disorder) were denied to a mother following the death of her son in a motor accident because her pathological grief reaction was not caused by the shock of the accident but was rather a consequence of later events, such as the acquittal of the driver who had crashed into her son on a charge of causing death by dangerous driving. Cf *Tredget v Bexley HA* [1994] 5 Med LR 178 (County Ct) in which damages for pathological grief reaction were awarded to a mother and father in respect of the traumatic birth, and death two days later, of their son caused by medical negligence. Bereavement damages, awarded pursuant to s 1A of the Fatal Accidents Act 1976, inserted by s 3(1) of the Administration of Justice Act 1982, differ because they do not depend on proof of any illness.

[21]   These examples were given by Brennan J in *Jaensch v Coffey* (1984) 155 CLR 549, 565, cited with approval by Lord Ackner in *Alcock v Chief Constable of South Yorkshire Police* [1992] 1 AC 310, 400. Contra is *Kralj v McGrath* [1986] 1 All ER 54 in which it appears that damages were awarded to a mother in respect of psychiatric injury attributable not to a single isolated shock, but to concern for her baby occurring over a period of eight weeks after which he died.

[22]   [1994] 2 WLR 554. See C Hilson, "Negligence and child abuse" (1994) 138 SJ 422. There has been an appeal to the House of Lords.

[23]   [1994] 2 WLR 554, 573. This is supported by *Walker v Northumberland CC* (1994) 144 NLJ 1659, see paras 2.49-2.50 below. See also *Campbelltown City Council v Mackay* (1989) 15 NSWLR 501, see para 2.44 n 138 below.

[24]   [1992] 1 AC 310, 400.

development of the law was to be expected and Lord Bridge in *McLoughlin*[25] had warned against the temptation of seeking to freeze the law in a rigid position. Secondly, the problem of "opening the door to claims by plaintiffs ever more remote from and ever more distantly related to the victims of the calamity",[26] did not arise in relation to this claim by the child. And thirdly, the harm was of the very type which the defendant psychiatrist should have been exercising her skill to try to prevent. Staughton and Peter Gibson LJJ struck out the child's claim in negligence without expressing any view on whether psychiatric illness which is not the result of a sudden occurrence is compensatable.

2.7 Sir Thomas Bingham MR's dissenting judgment was the subject of comment and clarification by the Court of Appeal in *Sion v Hampstead Health Authority*.[27] In that case a father stayed by his injured son's hospital bedside for fourteen days, watching him deteriorate in health and fall into a coma before finally dying. The plaintiff father alleged negligence on the part of the hospital staff in caring for his son, as a result of which he, the plaintiff, suffered psychiatric illness. It was argued for the plaintiff, based on the remarks of Sir Thomas Bingham MR in *Newham*, that it was unnecessary to prove a sudden or any shock. However the Court of Appeal, in upholding the striking out of the claim by Brooke J, disagreed and interpreted Sir Thomas Bingham MR's comments as being intended to apply only to a case like *Newham*, where the plaintiffs were primary, and not secondary, victims. It was firmly held that, subject to a change in the law by the House of Lords, the relevant psychiatric illness must be shock-induced where, as in the usual case, the claim involves secondary victims.

2.8 The requirement of a psychiatric illness that is, in general, shock-induced is relevant not only to determining whether a defendant is liable but also to *quantifying* damages. For having decided that there is a compensatable psychiatric illness the courts must award damages for that illness, and its consequences, alone and not for the non-compensatable mental distress or illness that the plaintiff may also have suffered. In *Hinz v Berry*,[28] the Court of Appeal considered an appeal against an award of £4,000 damages for shock-induced psychiatric illness. Lord Pearson identified five causes of the depressed state of the plaintiff: (1) grief and sorrow at losing her husband; (2) anxiety about the welfare of her injured children; (3) financial stress due to the loss of the family's bread-winner; (4) adjustment to a new life; and (5) shock of witnessing the accident.[29] Of the five, it was held that only the

---

[25] [1983] 1 AC 410, 443.

[26] [1994] 2 WLR 554, 573.

[27] Unreported, 27 May 1994, Transcript No QBENI 93/0122/E. Cf *Tredget v Bexley HA* [1994] 5 Med LR 178.

[28] [1970] 2 QB 40.

[29] *Ibid*, 44.

fifth was compensatable. In Lord Pearson's words, damages "should be only for that additional element which has been contributed by the shock of witnessing the accident, and which would not have occurred if she had not suffered that shock."[30] As Lord Denning MR put it, "[T]he court has to draw a line between sorrow and grief for which damages are not recoverable, and nervous shock and psychiatric illness for which damages are recoverable. The way to do this is to estimate how much [the plaintiff] would have suffered if, for instance, her husband had been killed in an accident when she was 50 miles away: and compare it with what she is now, having suffered all the shock due to being present at the accident."[31] In *Alcock*, Lord Oliver identified *Hinz v Berry* as "a useful illustration of the extreme difficulty of separating the compensatable injury arising from the presence of the plaintiff at the scene of an accident from the non-compensatable consequences flowing from the simple fact that the accident has occurred...."[32]

(2) It must have been reasonably foreseeable that the plaintiff might suffer a psychiatric illness as a result of the defendant's negligence.

2.9 In considering whether a duty of care is owed, it is material to consider what the defendant ought to have foreseen as a reasonable person.[33] "It is not every emotional disturbance or every shock which should have been foreseen."[34] The plaintiff must establish that the chain of causation between the defendant's negligence and the psychiatric illness, considered ex post facto in the light of all that has happened, was "reasonably foreseeable" by the "reasonable man".[35] The test has been described as undemanding,[36] and what must be established is that there was a "real" risk of psychiatric illness: the kind of risk which a reasonable person would not brush aside as far-fetched or fanciful.[37] In *Page v Smith*[38] the plaintiff had been directly involved in a car collision, but did not sustain any resulting physical injury. His claim for shock-induced psychiatric illness (a recurrence of myalgic encephalomyelitis (ME)) was rejected on appeal on the basis that a psychiatric illness was not reasonably

---

[30] *Ibid*, 45.

[31] *Ibid*, 43.

[32] [1992] 1 AC 310, 413. See also *Schneider v Eisovitch* [1960] 2 QB 430, 442 in which Paull J described the process of dividing up the consequences of the shock as "extremely difficult".

[33] *Bourhill v Young* [1943] AC 92, 101, *per* Lord Russell of Killowen.

[34] *Ibid*, 117, *per* Lord Porter.

[35] *McLoughlin v O'Brian* [1983] 1 AC 410, 432, *per* Lord Bridge.

[36] *Wyong Shire Council v Shirt* (1980) 146 CLR 40.

[37] *Ibid*, 44ff, *per* Mason J (referring to Lord Reid's judgment in *The Wagon Mound (No 2)* [1967] AC 617). See J Swanton, "Issues in Tort Liability for Nervous Shock" (1992) 66 ALJ 495, 501. See also P Vines, "Proximity as Principle or Category: Nervous Shock in Australia and England" (1993) 16 UNSWLJ 458, 462.

[38] [1994] 4 All ER 522. There has been an appeal to the House of Lords.

foreseeable in a person of ordinary fortitude as a result of a collision of moderate severity with some damage to the car but none to himself.[39] The court had in mind what may be a "reasonably possible result" of the event in question, "even if unlikely".[40] It was stressed that psychiatric injury was not of the same type as physical injury[41] and that "[f]oreseeability means foreseeability of damage caused by mental trauma. Foreseeability of physical injury is neither necessary nor sufficient".[42]

2.10   It is an important point that in applying the reasonable foreseeability test, and in the absence of special knowledge by the defendant to the contrary, the plaintiff is assumed to be a person of normal disposition and phlegm, or reasonable fortitude.[43] This requirement is intended to exclude from compensation those who are abnormally sensitive to psychiatric illness. However, once it is established that a person of reasonable fortitude might foreseeably have suffered psychiatric illness, the normal "eggshell skull" or "thin skull" rule of remoteness of damage applies, so that the plaintiff can recover for the full extent of the illness, even if it is exacerbated by a predisposition to mental illness or disorder.[44] So the tortfeasor need not compensate the exceptionally sensitive, but must compensate those who develop exceptionally severe illness because of their sensitivity if the negligence would have caused psychiatric illness in a normally robust individual.[45]

2.11   Lord Bridge in *McLoughlin*[46] thought that, in determining what was reasonably foreseeable, the judge could either "receive the evidence of psychiatrists as to the degree of probability that the particular cause would produce the particular effect, and apply to that the appropriate legal test of reasonable foreseeability as the criterion of the defendant's duty of care." Or, the judge, "relying on his own

---

[39]   *Ibid*, 544, 546-548, 552, 553.

[40]   *Ibid*, 544, *per* Ralph Gibson LJ.

[41]   *Ibid*, 548 and 550-552.

[42]   *Ibid*, 549, *per* Hoffmann LJ.

[43]   This requirement derives from the speeches of Lord Wright and Lord Porter in *Bourhill v Young* [1943] AC 92, 110, 117. See also, eg, Lord Russell of Killowen in *McLoughlin v O'Brian* [1983] 1 AC 410, 429. In *Page v Smith* [1994] 4 All ER 522 the Court of Appeal clarified that this requirement applies whether the plaintiff is involved in the accident (albeit not physically injured) or is an onlooker.

[44]   *Page v Smith* [1994] 4 All ER 522, 547, 549-550. See also *Brice v Brown* [1984] 1 All ER 997. Nor does it matter that the precise nature of the injury (or the precise psychiatric diagnosis) could not reasonably have been foreseen, although the plaintiff's pre-existing susceptibility may lead to a discount in the quantum of damages because of the chance that the illness would have been precipitated by other vicissitudes in the plaintiff's life in any event: *ibid*, 1007. T Weir, in his review of N J Mullany and P R Handford, *Tort Liability for Psychiatric Damage* (1993), criticises the equating of "thin skins and thin skulls": [1993] CLJ 520, 521.

[45]   See M A Jones, "'Ordinary shock' - thin skull rules O.K.?" (1984-1985) 4 Lit 114, 116-117.

[46]   [1983] 1 AC 410, 432.

opinion of the operation of cause and effect in psychiatric medicine, as fairly representative of that of the educated layman, should treat himself as the reasonable man and form his own view from the primary facts as to whether the proven chain of cause and effect was reasonably foreseeable." Not surprisingly, Lord Bridge ultimately preferred the second approach in the context of psychiatric illness[47] not only because all the authorities supported it but because it produced a degree of certainty,[48] whereas the opinions of medical practitioners might differ widely.[49]

(3) The plaintiff can recover if the foreseeable psychiatric illness arose from a reasonable fear of immediate physical injury to himself or herself.

2.12   As shown in the early leading case of *Dulieu v White*,[50] there is no difficulty where the psychiatric illness arises from the plaintiff's reasonable fear of immediate physical injury to himself or herself. In that case it was held that the plaintiff could recover for psychiatric illness because it had been brought on by fear for her own safety when the defendant negligently drove a horse-drawn van into a public house where she was standing behind the bar. The court rejected the Privy Council's decision in *Victorian Railways Commissioners v Coultas*[51] to the effect that "pure" psychiatric illness (that is, where there was no physical contact) was irrecoverable in the tort of negligence.

(4) Where the defendant has negligently injured or imperilled someone other than the plaintiff (but probably excluding the defendant himself or herself) and the plaintiff, as a result, has foreseeably suffered a shock-induced psychiatric illness, the plaintiff can recover if he or she can establish the requisite degree of proximity in terms of:

(a) the class of persons whose claims should be recognised and

---

[47] After saying that "[f]oreseeability, in any given set of circumstances, is ultimately a question of fact", Lord Bridge thought that, if a claim in negligence depended on whether a defect in a complicated piece of machinery was foreseeably a cause of injury, the judge would decide the question according to the expert evidence of engineers. But, unless the defendant were an engineer, that seems a controversial assertion. Reasonable foreseeability has been described as a difficult question of fact and law: J Williams, "Torts - Nervous Shock - Relation to Nominate Torts" (1968) 46 Can BR 515, 517.

[48] But see *Glasgow Corpn v Muir* [1943] AC 448, 457, *per* Lord Macmillan; J G Fleming, "Remoteness and Duty: The Control Devices in Liability for Negligence" (1953) 31 Can BR 471, 489; A L Goodhart, "Emotional Shock and the Unimaginative Taxicab Driver" (1953) 69 LQR 347, 350-351; P G Heffey, "The Negligent Infliction of Nervous Shock in Road and Industrial Accidents: Part I" (1974) 48 ALJ 196.

[49] However Lord Bridge also stressed that the judges must be informed by modern medical thinking.

[50] [1901] 2 KB 669.

[51] (1888) 13 App Cas 222.

(b) the closeness of the plaintiff to the accident in time and space and

(c) the means by which the shock is caused.

2.13 The restriction in *Dulieu v White* - that psychiatric illness was actionable but only if it arose from the plaintiff's reasonable fear for his or her own safety - was in turn departed from in *Hambrook v Stokes Bros*.[52] In that case a mother suffered "nervous shock" when realising that a runaway lorry might have injured her daughter whom she had just escorted round the bend in the road from which the lorry had come. But once such secondary victims were entitled to claim, the law inevitably had to face up to the difficulty of where to draw the line which demarcates those secondary victims who can claim from those who cannot. It is this central problem that continues to bedevil the law and with which this paper is primarily concerned.

2.14 Prior to the decision in *Alcock*,[53] there was disagreement as to whether the relevant line should be drawn by simply asking, as with any other personal injury, whether the defendant should have reasonably foreseen that his conduct might cause the plaintiff shock-induced psychiatric illness; or, whether, on the contrary, shock-induced psychiatric illness should be treated more restrictively than any other personal injury by insisting on limitations over and above the test of reasonable foreseeability.

→ perhaps needed more fleshing out?

2.15 In *McLoughlin*[54] the House was divided. Lord Scarman and Lord Bridge (and probably also Lord Russell of Killowen) thought that the test of reasonable foreseeability was the sole test for determining whether there is a duty of care on the part of the defendant. Factors such as spatial, physical and temporal proximity, and the relationship of the plaintiff to the immediate victim of the accident were important as bearing on the degree of foreseeability of the plaintiff's psychiatric illness. However, neither Lord Scarman nor Lord Bridge thought that these represented legal limitations or hard and fast lines of policy.[55]

---

[52] [1925] 1 KB 141. See para 2.32 below.

[53] [1992] 1 AC 310.

[54] [1983] 1 AC 410.

[55] [1983] 1 AC 410, 431, 441-443 respectively. "[I]f asked where the thing is to stop," said Lord Bridge, "I should answer, in an adaptation of the language of Lord Wright...and Stephenson LJ... 'where in the particular case the good sense of the judge, enlightened by progressive awareness of mental illness, decides'": *ibid*, 443. Similarly, Lord Russell of Killowen gave no express guidance on how the reasonable foreseeability test should be applied, for "to attempt in advance solutions, or even guidelines, in hypothetical cases may well...in this field, do more harm than good": *ibid*, 429. Where appropriate, the "reasonably foreseeable test" must be applied "untrammelled by spatial, physical or temporal limits": *ibid*, 431, *per* Lord Scarman.

2.16   Lord Wilberforce, on the other hand, (with whom Lord Edmund-Davies agreed) thought that reasonable foreseeability was not the sole test in determining the existence of a duty of care and that in cases of psychiatric illness there should be overriding limitations on the principle of liability for reasonably foreseeable harm. The limitations related to three elements inherent in a "nervous shock" claim: the class of persons whose claims should be recognised; the proximity of such persons to the accident; and the means by which the shock is caused. Lord Wilberforce said that, although not excluded, relationships other than parent-child or spouse must be very carefully scrutinised. "The closer the tie (not merely in relationship, but in care) the greater the claim for consideration. The claim, in any case, has to be judged in the light of the other factors, such as proximity to the scene in time and place, and the nature of the accident."[56] He said that the claims of ordinary bystanders were not recognised by existing law and that he thought this position justified.[57] As regards proximity to the accident, he thought that this must be close in both time and space. To insist on direct aural or visual perception, however, would be impractical and unjust, and under the 'immediate aftermath' doctrine, one who came very soon on the scene should not be excluded. This extension was confined to those of whom it could be said that one could expect nothing else than that he or she would come immediately to the scene (normally a parent or a spouse).[58] Lastly, as regards communication, Lord Wilberforce thought that it was right that the law should not compensate shock brought about by communication by a third party. However, he believed that consideration might have to be given to whether communication that is an equivalent of sight or hearing, for example through simultaneous television, sufficed.[59]

2.17   It is difficult to discern a clear ratio in *McLoughlin*, and the subsequent cases prior to *Alcock* did not clarify which of the two approaches should be adopted.[60] However, the position has now been resolved by the decision of the House of Lords in *Alcock*. All five of their Lordships in that case endorsed the approach of Lord Wilberforce in *McLoughlin*. Thus, in addition to reasonable foreseeability, the right to recover

---

[56] *Ibid*, 422.

[57] *Ibid*.

[58] *Ibid*.

[59] *Ibid*, 423.

[60] *Brice v Brown* [1984] 1 All ER 997, 1006 and *Wigg v British Railways Board, The Times* 4 February 1986, appear to have regarded the test and fundamental question as one of reasonable foreseeability *simpliciter*. But in *Attia v British Gas Plc* [1988] QB 304, 319-320, Bingham LJ thought that the discernible majority ratio in *McLoughlin v O'Brian* was that reasonable foreseeability was a necessary but not sufficient condition of liability: policy might preclude recovery of foreseeable shock. In *Ravenscroft v Rederiaktiebølaget Transatlantic* [1991] 3 All ER 73, 84-85 Ward J thought that in addition to reasonable foreseeability, proximity must also be established such as rendered it fair, just and reasonable that liability be imposed. Cf *Ravenscroft v Rederiaktiebølaget Transatlantic (Note)* [1992] 2 All ER 470 (CA).

damages for shock-induced psychiatric injury must be decided according to the three tests of "proximity" identified by Lord Wilberforce.

2.18 Before turning to a detailed examination of those proximity tests, we outline the position in *Alcock*. Claims were brought by sixteen relatives and friends of spectators involved in the disaster at the Hillsborough football stadium. It was admitted that the deaths and injuries of the primary victims occurred as a result of negligence by the police and it was assumed for the purposes of the case that each of the plaintiffs had proved the infliction of psychiatric illness.[61] Ten of the plaintiffs succeeded at trial but the Court of Appeal allowed the defendant's appeal in respect of nine of those successful plaintiffs and dismissed cross-appeals by the six unsuccessful plaintiffs.[62] Ten of the fifteen plaintiffs unsuccessfully appealed to the House of Lords. Of these, Brian Harrison, who lost both his brothers, and Robert Alcock, who lost his brother-in-law, were both present at the match. Brian Harrison had stayed up all night and was informed about the deaths the next morning, and Robert Alcock searched until about midnight when he identified the body in the temporary mortuary. None of the other eight plaintiffs were present at the match. Six of them watched the events unfold on live television: Harold and Agnes Copoc, who lost their son, Harold Copoc later travelling to Sheffield to identify the body; Brenda Hennessy, who lost her brother; Denise Hough, who also lost a brother, whose body she identified two days later; Stephen Jones, who lost his brother; and Alexandra Penk, who lost her fiancé. The remaining two - Catherine Jones, who lost a brother, and Joseph Kehoe, who lost his grandson - heard of events from friends or on the radio and later watched scenes of the disaster on recorded television.

2.19 The House of Lords held that in the cases of the two plaintiffs who had been present at the match the necessary close tie of love and affection had not been proved and could not be presumed for brothers or brothers-in-law; and in the cases of the other eight the viewing of the disaster on television or viewing the bodies in the mortuary could not be said to be equivalent to being within sight and hearing of the event or its immediate aftermath. William Pemberton, the plaintiff who succeeded at trial, and in respect of whom the defendant did not appeal, was a father who had travelled with his son to the match, stayed on the coach, watched the events as they happened on its television and searched for his son until he identified him in the temporary mortuary.

---

[61] [1992] 1 AC 310, 318 (Hidden J); 351 (Parker LJ); 406 (Lord Oliver).

[62] For a detailed account of the position of the unsuccessful appellants, see [1992] 1 AC 310, 352-355 (Parker LJ), quoted by Lord Keith at pp 393-394, and for the position of the successful plaintiff, see *ibid*, 339, 344.

(a) The class of persons whose claims should be recognised

Persons with a tie of love and affection to the primary victim

2.20 The affirmation in the Hillsborough case that proximity is an independent requirement restricting the test of reasonable foreseeability may operate to limit the availability of damages for psychiatric illness. However, in one respect, namely the class of persons entitled to claim damages, the decision may lead to the widening of liability.

2.21 Although recovery for shock-induced psychiatric illness had not previously been limited expressly to those within a marital or parental relationship with the primary victim, in almost all the reported cases[63] successful claimants (other than rescuers or involuntary participants)[64] did fall within one of these categories. In *Alcock*, however, the House of Lords made it clear that the crucial factor was the *quality* of the relationship and the necessary relationship was to be proved by reference to the strength of the bonds of love and affection between the parties, not by reference to a particular blood or marital tie.[65] There was general agreement that the class of potential plaintiffs could not be tightly defined; to attempt to do so, or to draw a dividing line between one degree of relationship and another, would be arbitrary and illogical.[66] Lord Oliver stated that to postulate rigid categories of relationship within which claims might succeed, but outside which they were necessarily doomed to failure, would work great injustice and could not be rationally justified.[67] Hence distant relatives and close friends may in principle succeed.

2.22 The closeness of the tie must be proved by the plaintiff, although this can be rebuttably presumed[68] in the case of parents, children and spouses.[69] Lord Keith thought that the requisite proximity could also be presumed in the case of a

---

[63] An exception, albeit covered by proposition (5), not (4), is *Owens v Liverpool Corpn* [1939] 1 KB 394, in which the plaintiffs included an uncle, cousin and husband of the cousin of a deceased person whose coffin was overturned.

[64] Paras 2.26-2.28 below.

[65] [1992] 1 AC 310, 397, *per* Lord Keith; 403-404, *per* Lord Ackner; 415-416, *per* Lord Oliver; 422, *per* Lord Jauncey. This emphasis on the quality of the relationship was also put forward by Lord Wilberforce in *McLoughlin v O'Brian* [1983] 1 AC 410, 422. See B Lynch, "A Victory for Pragmatism? Nervous Shock Reconsidered" (1992) 108 LQR 367, 369.

[66] *Alcock v Chief Constable of South Yorkshire Police* [1992] 1 AC 310, 422, *per* Lord Jauncey.

[67] *Ibid*, 415.

[68] The presumption is rebuttable because a mother who handed over her child at birth and has never seen it since, or a husband and wife who have been parted for years and hate each other, should not have a better claim than strangers: [1992] 1 AC 310, 359-360, *per* Parker LJ.

[69] [1992] 1 AC 310, 397-398, *per* Lord Keith; 403, *per* Lord Ackner; 422, *per* Lord Jauncey. See also [1992] 1 AC 310, 359-361, *per* Parker LJ, and 376, *per* Stocker LJ.

fiancé(e).[70] However, their Lordships did not consider that such a presumption was raised between grandparent and grandchild or between siblings; "The quality of brotherly love is well known to differ widely - from Cain and Abel to David and Jonathan."[71] The content of the proof required in relation to distant relatives and friends was not articulated in *Alcock* beyond it being said that their love and affection for the victim should be "comparable to that of the normal parent, spouse or child of the victim".[72] It is doubtful whether this was meant to import more than that the tie of love and affection must be a close and not a fleeting or distant one, but Mullany and Handford read more into this by questioning whether it is sensible for "the bond between friends or cousins, for example, [to] be assessed by reference to the most formal relationships."[73]

So why not brothers etc?

Persons with no tie of love and affection to the primary victim
(i) Bystanders

2.23   In *Bourhill v Young*[74] Lord Porter stated that:

> "The driver of a car or vehicle, even though careless, is entitled to assume that the ordinary frequenter of the streets has sufficient fortitude to endure such incidents as may from time to time be expected to occur in them...and is not to be considered negligent towards one who does not possess the customary phlegm."[75]

Similarly, in *McLoughlin* Lord Wilberforce considered that the law's denial of claims by ordinary bystanders was justified, either on the basis that such persons must be presumed to be possessed of fortitude sufficient to enable them to endure the calamities of modern life or on the basis that defendants cannot be expected to compensate the world at large.[76]

2.24   Although it was accepted in *Alcock* that a mere bystander could not ordinarily recover, there are dicta indicating that in exceptional circumstances this might be possible. Lord Keith stated that a bystander might recover "if the circumstances of

---

[70]   [1992] 1 AC 310, 398.

[71]   *Alcock v Chief Constable of South Yorkshire Police* [1992] 1 AC 310, 406, *per* Lord Ackner.

[72]   [1992] 1 AC 310, 403, *per* Lord Ackner. See also at p 422, *per* Lord Jauncey.

[73]   N J Mullany and P R Handford, *Tort Liability for Psychiatric Damage* (1993) p 126.

[74]   [1943] AC 92.

[75]   *Ibid*, 117. Lord Porter did intimate later in his speech, however, (at p 120) that if the noise of the collision had been exceptionally loud or if the plaintiff had witnessed a particularly gruesome accident, damages might have been recoverable. In fact the plaintiff's claim in *Bourhill* was rejected by the majority not because claims by bystanders are necessarily doomed, but rather because, in the circumstances, the injury to her was not reasonably foreseeable.

[76]   [1983] 1 AC 410, 422.

a catastrophe occurring very close to him were particularly horrific."[77] In terms reminiscent of Lord Porter in *Bourhill v Young,* Lord Oliver spoke of circumstances of such horror as would be "likely to traumatise even the most phlegmatic spectator",[78] and Lord Ackner of circumstances such that "a reasonably strong-nerved person would have been so shocked".[79] However those dicta were rejected by the Court of Appeal in *McFarlane v EE Caledonia Ltd*[80] in refusing damages for psychiatric illness to a witness to the Piper Alpha oil rig disaster in which 164 men died. Stuart-Smith LJ, with whom McCowan and Ralph Gibson LJJ agreed, said: "In my judgment both as a matter of principle and policy the court should not extend the duty to those who are mere bystanders or witnesses of horrific events unless there is a sufficient degree of proximity, which requires both nearness in time and place and a close relationship of love and affection between plaintiff and victim".[81]

2.25 Even if in exceptional circumstances bystanders were able to recover, those who choose to come to the scene of an accident because of morbid curiosity cannot recover on the grounds that their choice falls within the doctrine of *volenti non fit injuria* or amounts to a *novus actus interveniens.*[82]

(ii) Rescuers

2.26 It has long been established that a defendant owes a duty of care not only to those who are directly threatened or injured by his or her careless acts, but also to those who, as a result, are induced reasonably to go to their rescue and suffer physical injury in so doing. As was recognised by Cardozo J in *Wagner v International Railway Co,*

> "Danger invites rescue. The cry of distress is the summons to relief. The law does not ignore these reactions of the mind in tracing conduct to its consequences. It recognises them as normal. It places their effects within the range of the natural and probable. The wrong that imperils

---

[77] [1992] 1 AC 310, 397.

[78] *Ibid,* 416.

[79] *Ibid,* 403. Lord Ackner considered that in principle damages could not be ruled out where, for example, a petrol tanker careered out of control into a school in session and burst into flames causing a shocked passer-by to suffer psychiatric illness: [1992] 1 AC 310, 403. Lord Bridge in *McLoughlin* gave the example of a passenger in a train involved in a rail disaster, uninjured and in no way involved in the rescue operations, but witnessing the terrible carnage while he waited for transport to take him home: [1983] 1 AC 410, 442-443.

[80] [1994] 2 All ER 1; noted by Tan Keng Feng, "Nervous Shock: Bystander Witnessing a Catastrophe" (1995) 111 LQR 48. See also para 2.26 below.

[81] [1994] 2 All ER 1, 14.

[82] *Jaensch v Coffey* (1984) 155 CLR 549, 570, *per* Brennan J.

life is a wrong to the imperilled victim; it is a wrong also to his rescuer."[83]

It is generally accepted that the provision of a remedy for rescuers reflects the desire, as a matter of policy, not to discourage their activities. In *Chadwick v British Railways Board*[84] this principle was extended to the psychiatric consequences of rescue attempts,[85] and its application in this context was approved by Lord Wilberforce in *McLoughlin*.[86] The limits of the principle are illustrated by *Rapley v P & O European Ferries (Dover) Ltd*.[87] In that case the plaintiff was not present when the catastrophe occurred but he went to the scene as a volunteer three days later and helped the relatives of those injured, but not the injured themselves. The Court of Appeal distinguished *Chadwick* and held that the plaintiff could not be described as a rescuer in ordinary terms. Similarly, in *McFarlane v EE Caledonia Ltd*[88] the plaintiff failed in his submission that he was entitled to recover for psychiatric illness sustained in the capacity of rescuer because his involvement in the rescue operations had been very limited.[89] He had been assisting the rescue operations at the Piper Alpha disaster, but he had been on a rescue vessel which had not come closer than 100 metres to the burning platform, and his active involvement was limited to moving blankets, helping to clear space for the reception of casualties, and meeting, and possibly helping, two walking casualties. This was held to be insufficient to bring him within the "rescuer" category.

[83] (1921) 232 NY 176, 180. A similar principle was adopted by the English Court of Appeal in *Haynes v Harwood* [1935] 1 KB 146.

[84] [1967] 1 WLR 912.

[85] The plaintiff recovered damages for psychiatric illness sustained as a result of his prolonged rescue efforts at the scene of a serious railway accident which had occurred near his home in which ninety persons were killed and bodies and injured passengers were trapped in the wreckage. The shock was caused neither by fear for his own safety nor for that of close relations. Waller J dealt with the case on the basis that it was the horror of the whole experience which caused his reaction: *ibid*, 918.

[86] [1983] 1 AC 410, 419. In *Alcock* [1992] 1 AC 310, 408, 420-421 Lords Oliver and Jauncey recognised that the "rescue" cases were well established.

[87] Unreported, 21 February 1991 (CA). See N J Mullany and P R Handford, *Tort Liability for Psychiatric Damage* (1993) pp 110-111.

[88] [1994] 2 All ER 1. See para 2.24 above.

[89] *Ibid*, 12-13, *per* Stuart-Smith LJ (McCowan and Ralph Gibson LJJ concurring).

2.27   In the case of *physical* injury it is no answer to a claim by a *professional* rescuer, such as a fireman, that this is within the ordinary risk of his or her occupation.[90] The point does not appear to have been decided upon by the courts in the context of psychiatric illness, but it is likely that the same rule applies to psychiatric illness sustained in the course of a professional rescue operation.[91]

(iii) Involuntary participants

2.28   In *Dooley v Cammell Laird & Co Ltd*[92] a crane driver suffered shock-induced psychiatric illness when he saw a rope snap and a load from his crane fall into the hold of a ship where he knew fellow workers were unloading. He recovered damages even though no-one was in fact harmed. In *Alcock* this sort of case was rationalised on the basis that the plaintiff has been "intimately"[93] or "personally"[94] involved in the shocking event out of which the action arises. And Lord Oliver said that this category covered cases "where the negligent act of the defendant has put the plaintiff in the position of being, or of thinking that he is about to be or has been, the involuntary cause of another's death or injury and the illness complained of stems from the shock to the plaintiff of the consciousness of this supposed fact."[95]

(b) Closeness of the plaintiff to the accident in time and space[96]

2.29   The plaintiff must be close to the accident in time and space. This requirement is obviously satisfied where the plaintiff is present at the accident. But the courts have

---

[90]   *Ogwo v Taylor* [1988] AC 431 (HL); *Salmon v Seafarer Restaurants Ltd* [1983] 1 WLR 1264. In contrast, the fact that members of the emergency services are in a sense employed to take risks has led some American courts to deny liability to them on the part of the person whose negligence creates the danger. This has been called the "fireman's rule". See *Krauth v Geller* (1960) 157 A 2d 129, 130-131 (Supreme Court of New Jersey); *Walters v Sloan* (1977) 571 P 2d 609 (Supreme Court of California); *Winfield and Jolowicz on Tort* (14th ed 1994) p 739; J Fleming, *The Law of Torts* (8th ed 1992) p 454.

[91]   In *Hale v London Underground Ltd* [1993] PIQR Q30 liability was admitted in the case of a professional fireman who sustained post-traumatic stress disorder in the King's Cross fire. Out-of-court settlements have been reached with police officers on duty at Hillsborough who carried out rescue work and sustained post-traumatic stress disorder: see *The Times* 4 February 1995, p 9.

[92]   [1951] 1 Lloyd's Rep 271.

[93]   *Alcock v Chief Constable of South Yorkshire Police* [1992] 1 AC 310, 420, *per* Lord Jauncey.

[94]   *Ibid*, 408, *per* Lord Oliver.

[95]   *Ibid*. (Lord Oliver had in mind *Dooley v Cammell Laird & Co Ltd* [1951] 1 Lloyd's Rep 271, *Galt v British Railways Board* (1983) 133 NLJ 870, and *Wigg v British Railways Board, The Times* 4 February 1986). Lord Jauncey thought this category was "special": [1992] 1 AC 310, 420.

[96]   It has been suggested that the requirement of proximity in time and space could be combined with the requirement of direct sensory perception to form one "sight or sound" test: P Duff, "Criminal Injuries Compensation, Nervous Shock and Secondary Victims" (1992) 32 SLT 311, 312. See also M Davie, "Negligently Inflicted Psychiatric Illness: The Hillsborough Case in the House of Lords" (1992) 43 NILQ 237, 240; K J Nasir, "Nervous Shock and *Alcock*: The Judicial Buck Stops Here" (1992) 55 MLR 705, 708-709.

extended physical proximity to include the case where the plaintiff perceives the "immediate aftermath" of an accident. In *McLoughlin* the House of Lords held that it was not necessary for the plaintiff to perceive the accident itself. What was required was "a direct perception of some of the events which go to make up the accident as an entire event, and this includes seeing the immediate aftermath of the accident".[97] On the facts of that case the "immediate aftermath" extended to the hospital where the injured relatives were taken as a result of the accident. At the time of the accident the plaintiff was at her home about two miles away. An hour or so afterwards she was told of the accident and driven to the hospital, where she was informed that her youngest daughter was dead. She found her husband and two of her other children in a state of acute distress, still awaiting treatment and covered in oil and mud, in much the same state as they had been by the roadside. Lord Wilberforce and Lord Edmund-Davies drew an analogy between the facts in *McLoughlin* and the position of a rescuer such as the plaintiff in *Chadwick v British Railways Board*.[98] If a rescuer could recover when, acting in accordance with normal and irresistible human instinct, and indeed moral compulsion, he or she went to the scene of an accident, why could not a mother recover if, acting under the same motives, she went to the place to which her family had been taken?[99] It would be impractical and unjust, in Lord Wilberforce's view, to insist on direct and immediate sight or hearing of the accident. A person who was close to the scene and arrived there very soon after the accident should not be excluded.

2.30 The courts have tended to take a narrow view of what constitutes "the immediate aftermath". In *Alcock* several of the plaintiffs saw the bodies of their relatives in a temporary mortuary for the purposes of identification. Lord Ackner considered that, although it was clear from *McLoughlin* that subsequent identification might in principle fall within the "immediate aftermath", on the facts there was insufficient proximity in time and space to the accident.[100] In the earliest of the identification cases Mr Alcock had identified his brother-in-law in the mortuary some eight hours

---

97 [1983] 1 AC 410, 422 (Lord Wilberforce), citing with approval the Australian case of *Benson v Lee* [1972] VR 879, 880.

98 [1967] 1 WLR 912. See para 2.26 above.

99 [1983] 1 AC 410, 419, *per* Lord Wilberforce. See also *ibid*, 422, 424. The use of the "rescue" analogy in these circumstances has been questioned, however. Teff says that it is only because physical proximity to the scene of the accident has loomed so large as a criterion of liability that "judges may feel constrained to resort to artificial analogies such as rescue when such proximity is absent": "Liability for Negligently Inflicted Nervous Shock" (1983) 99 LQR 100, 110. On the matter of the plaintiff's motive, see para 2.30 below.

100 [1992] 1 AC 310, 404-405. Their Lordships' decision in *Alcock* on this point must cast doubt upon the first instance decision (unreported) in *Radford v Midland Red (West) Ltd* (1991) (cited in C Pugh and M Trimble, "Psychiatric Injury after Hillsborough" (1993) 163 British Journal of Psychiatry 425, 428). In that case Hodgson J awarded the plaintiff damages for psychiatric illness notwithstanding he did not arrive at the hospital until a couple of hours after the accident and in fact only saw his wife's body a day or two later following the hospital's advice.

after the accident: even if this could be described as part of the aftermath, it could not be described as part of the *immediate* aftermath. Lord Jauncey went further: the visits to the mortuary were outside the immediate aftermath of the disaster not only because of the time at which they were made but because of their *purpose*, namely identification as opposed to rescue or comfort.[101]

2.31   In *Taylor v Somerset Health Authority*[102] the deceased died from a heart attack, the final consequence of a progressively deteriorating heart condition which the defendants had negligently failed to diagnose. His widow, the plaintiff, went to the hospital within an hour of death and 20 minutes later was told of his death by a doctor. Shortly afterwards she visited the hospital mortuary, partly to identify the body but also because she could not believe what she had been told. Auld J held that the facts did not fall within the "immediate aftermath": rather, the shock was brought about by being told of the death. The primary purpose of the plaintiff's visit to the mortuary was to settle her disbelief, and this went to the fact of the death as distinct from the circumstances in which death came about. In addition, the court placed emphasis on the fact that the body bore no marks or signs of the sort which would have conjured up for her the circumstances of the death.[103] Again, in *Taylorson v Shieldness Produce Ltd*,[104] the Court of Appeal rejected the claims of the parents of the deceased on the basis, inter alia,[105] that the immediate aftermath did not extend to witnessing the deteriorating condition of their son following post-accident treatment. The parents had been informed of a serious accident to their son soon after it occurred and went straightaway to the hospital to which he had been admitted. They glimpsed their son briefly as he was being rushed to the intensive care unit. However, neither was allowed to see him again until some time after treatment (in the mother's case, some 24 hours after the accident).

2.32   What if the plaintiff does not see the accident, or its immediate aftermath, but merely sees something (for example, a runaway vehicle) which indicates that there

---

[101] [1992] 1 AC 310, 424. See also Lord Oliver at pp 416-417. Lord Jauncey's reference to the purpose of the visit to the mortuary may have been prompted by Lord Wilberforce's dicta in *McLoughlin v O'Brian* comparing a mother's motive to that of a rescuer: see para 2.29 above.

[102] [1993] PIQR P262. For a discussion of the decision in *Taylor* see R English, "Nervous Shock: Before the Aftermath" [1993] CLJ 204.

[103] Auld J's alternative ground for disallowing the claim was that, although the psychiatric illness was shock-induced, it had not been the consequence of a violent and sudden event. But this ground of reasoning was rejected by the Court of Appeal in *Sion v Hampstead Health Authority* (unreported, 27 May 1994, Transcript No QBENI 93/0122/E): see the judgment of Peter Gibson LJ at pp 25-26 of the transcript. See also para 2.7 above.

[104] [1994] PIQR P329. Cf *Kralj v McGrath* [1986] 1 All ER 54, 60-64: see para 2.5 n 21 above.

[105] The Court of Appeal also held that the psychiatric illness to the parents resulted from grief and not shock.

has just been an accident? In *Hambrook v Stokes Bros*[106] a mother did not see the accident in which her daughter was seriously injured. The mother had just escorted her three children part of the way to their school. Within a few yards of leaving her they turned a bend out of sight. Moments later, a runaway lorry knocked down her daughter, came round the bend and ran into a house. The mother became very anxious for the safety of her children, ran to search for them and eventually found her daughter in hospital. Liability was based on the mother's apprehension of danger to her daughter at the moment the lorry went by her, and counsel expressly disclaimed any suggestion that the plaintiff's injury was either due to or aggravated by her finding that her daughter was missing from school or by tracing her to, and seeing her in, hospital.[107] Given that there was a close relationship to the primary victim, and that the mother's shock had been occasioned through her own unaided senses, and that she was close to the accident in time and space, it did not matter that the shock was occasioned by a reasonable fear that others had already been injured.[108] As the plaintiff need only perceive circumstances suggesting peril it is also the case that, unlike the facts in *Hambrook v Stokes*, there may be no primary victim in fact.[109]

(c) The means by which the shock is caused (ie the requirement of perception through one's own unaided senses)

Third party communication

2.33   In *McLoughlin* Lord Wilberforce stated that the shock must come through sight or hearing of the event or its immediate aftermath. He also said that it was surely right that there should be no liability where the plaintiff's shock resulted from being told of the accident or event by a third party.[110] This was accepted in *Alcock*,[111] which cast doubt on, while not expressly overruling, the correctness of two earlier decisions, *Hevican v Ruane*[112] and *Ravenscroft v Rederiaktiebølaget Transatlantic*.[113] In *Hevican*, the plaintiff suffered clinical depression after his son was killed in a minibus crash. The plaintiff had been told about the accident by a friend of his son's, and was subsequently told of his son's death by the police. Mantell J, relying on Lord Bridge's speech in *McLoughlin*, held that the plaintiff was entitled to

---

[106]   [1925] 1 KB 141. The mother had died and the action was brought by her husband under the Fatal Accidents Act 1846.

[107]   [1925] 1 KB 141, 160.

[108]   See also Lord Porter in *Bourhill v Young* [1943] AC 92, 120.

[109]   *Dooley v Cammell Laird & Co Ltd* [1951] 1 Lloyd's Rep 271; and dicta by Lord Oliver in *Alcock* [1992] 1 AC 310, 412. Cf, however, 417 (Lord Oliver).

[110]   [1983] 1 AC 410, 423. See also *Bourhill v Young* 1941 SC 395, 399, *per* Lord Robertson.

[111]   [1992] 1 AC 310, 398, 400-401, 411, 417, 418.

[112]   [1991] 3 All ER 65.

[113]   [1991] 3 All ER 73.

damages notwithstanding that he was not present at the immediate aftermath of the accident and the shock was administered to him indirectly by a third party, on the basis that each link in the chain of causation was foreseeable. A similar conclusion was reached by Ward J in *Ravenscroft* on a similar set of facts. The decision in *Ravenscroft* has since been reversed by the Court of Appeal[114] on the ground that it could not stand alongside *Alcock*.

2.34　The earlier decision in *Schneider v Eisovitch*[115] may also need reconsideration. In that case the plaintiff, who was rendered unconscious in a car accident in which her husband was killed, was told of her husband's death when she regained consciousness in hospital. Paull J held that she could recover damages for psychiatric illness as well as for the physical injuries she sustained in the accident. Although she did not see her husband killed because she was unconscious, the news of his death which was conveyed to her later "was a consequence which flowed directly from the breach of duty towards the plaintiff".[116] Arguably this is inconsistent with the denial of damages to a person who suffers shock on hearing of the death or injury without being at the scene.[117]

[handwritten: → A duty to P: what consequences?]

2.35　It has been argued in support of *Schneider*, however, that it seems arbitrary and unfair to compensate a plaintiff who is less seriously injured and remains conscious and witnesses what happens to the other victims, while depriving one whose own injuries are so severe as to render her or him insensible. In addition, limiting damages for shock suffered in this way to those who have already been physically injured in an accident will not lead to an increase in the total number of claims.[118]

Live television broadcast

2.36　In *McLoughlin* Lord Wilberforce left open the question whether a simultaneous television broadcast qualified as direct perception of the accident or its immediate aftermath.[119] This issue was addressed in *Alcock*. The House of Lords agreed that

---

[114]　[1992] 2 All ER 470 (Note). See also *Taylor v Somerset Health Authority* [1993] PIQR P262, P267-P268 in which the rule precluding recovery for psychiatric injury induced by shock brought about by communication by a third party was followed.

[115]　[1960] 2 QB 430.

[116]　*Ibid*, 442.

[117]　J A Jolowicz, "Damages - Nervous Shock - Volunteer's Expenses" [1960] CLJ 156, 157-158; H Luntz, *Assessment of Damages for Personal Injury and Death* (3rd ed 1990) para 2.4.3. It has also been suggested that *Schneider v Eisovitch* is no longer supportable since it proceeded on the basis of the "direct consequences" test of remoteness which was overruled by the foreseeability test laid down in *The Wagon Mound* [1961] AC 388. But cf *Andrews v Williams* [1967] VR 831; *Kohn v State Government Insurance Commission* (1976) 15 SASR 255; *Kwok v British Columbia Ferry Corpn* (1987) 20 BCLR (2d) 318 which held that nothing in *The Wagon Mound* prevented *Schneider v Eisovitch* from applying in similar circumstances.

[118]　J Swanton, "Issues in Tort Liability for Nervous Shock" (1992) 66 ALJ 495, 500-501.

[119]　[1983] 1 AC 410, 423.

on the facts of that case the necessary degree of proximity was lacking, and that watching the Hillsborough scenes on television could not be equated with being within sight or hearing of the disaster or its aftermath.

2.37   A number of different reasons for this conclusion were advanced. Three of the five law lords (Lords Keith, Ackner and Jauncey) emphasised the fact that the television authorities had observed the broadcasting code of ethics which prohibited the transmission of scenes depicting the suffering of recognisable individuals.[120] The defendant was reasonably entitled to expect that this code would be observed and it was therefore not reasonably foreseeable that the plaintiffs would sustain psychiatric injury.[121] Lords Keith and Oliver also considered that, because death and suffering by recognisable individuals were not depicted, it was not reasonably foreseeable that the scenes would give rise to shock, as opposed to grave concern and worry.[122] Lord Jauncey also thought that watching the televised scenes could not be equated with actually seeing or hearing of the event or its immediate aftermath because "a television programme such as that transmitted from Hillsborough involves cameras at different viewpoints showing scenes all of which no one individual would see, edited pictures and a commentary superimposed."[123]

2.38   Although the tenor of their Lordships' speeches in *Alcock* was generally unfavourable to recovery for psychiatric illness sustained through the medium of television, Lord Ackner and Lord Oliver expressed the opinion that witnessing actual injury to the primary victim on simultaneous television might in some cases be the equivalent to actually seeing or hearing the event or its immediate aftermath and thus suffice. They both adverted to the example given by Nolan LJ in the Court of Appeal of a publicity seeking organisation arranging for the simultaneous broadcast of a balloon trip made by a number of children. Whilst filming and transmitting pictures of the event the cameras showed the balloon suddenly bursting into flames.[124] Lord Ackner thought many other such situations could be imagined where the impact of the simultaneous television pictures would be as great as, if not greater than, the actual sight of the accident.[125] In such situations those with a sufficiently close relationship to the primary victim might be able to recover for their shock-induced psychiatric illness.

---

[120]   [1992] 1 AC 310, 398, *per* Lord Keith (with whom Lord Oliver, 417, agreed); 405, *per* Lord Ackner; 423, *per* Lord Jauncey.

[121]   Counsel for the plaintiffs accepted that had the code been breached this would have been a "novus actus" breaking the chain of causation: *ibid*, 405.

[122]   [1992] 1 AC 310, 398, 417.

[123]   *Ibid*, 423. See also Parker LJ in the Court of Appeal: *ibid*, 362-363. See B McDonald, "Negligence - Duty of Care - Nervous Shock" (1992) 66 ALJ 386, 387.

[124]   [1992] 1 AC 310, 405, *per* Lord Ackner; 417, *per* Lord Oliver; 386-387, *per* Nolan LJ. Lord Jauncey left the question open: *ibid*, 423.

[125]   *Ibid*, 405.

Recorded television and radio broadcast

2.39 Some of the plaintiffs in the Hillsborough case suffered psychiatric illness as a result of hearing the news on the radio or seeing recorded television footage of the tragedy. If a claimant watching a *simultaneous* television broadcast did not satisfy the requirement of proximity, it followed *a fortiori* that a claimant who listened to the radio or saw a subsequent television recording could not recover.[126]

(d) Where the primary victim is the defendant (ie self-inflicted injury)

2.40 Although there is no English decision on this point, a dictum by Lord Robertson in his judgment in the Court of Session in *Bourhill v Young*[127] suggests that damages are not recoverable where the defendant's injury is self-inflicted on the basis that there must be an end at some reasonable point to the legal consequences of a careless act.[128] The same opinion was expressed by Deane J in *Jaensch v Coffey*.[129] He said, "[O]n the present state of the law, such a duty of care will not exist unless the reasonably foreseeable psychiatric injury was sustained as a result of the death, injury or peril of someone other than the person whose carelessness is alleged to have caused the injury...[It] is unnecessary to determine whether [this limitation] is properly to be seen as part of the requirement of proximity of relationship or as constituting some other and special controlling rule based on policy considerations. As at present advised, I am inclined to see [it] as [a] necessary criterion of the existence of the requisite proximity of relationship in the sense that, for policy reasons, the relationship will not be adjudged as being 'so' close 'as' to give rise to a duty of care unless [it] be satisfied."

2.41 Although the question did not fall to be determined in *Alcock*, Lord Oliver cited Deane J and suspected that an English court would be likely to take a similar view.[130]

---

[126] *Ibid*, 423, *per* Lord Jauncey.

[127] 1941 SC 395, 399. This also seems to be the law in Canada and Germany: see Appendix, paras 32 and 48 below.

[128] See, however, *A v B's Trustees* 1906 13 SLT 830; see Appendix, para 4 below.

[129] (1984) 155 CLR 549, 604. For other Australian cases on this point see Appendix, para 12 n 45 below.

[130] [1992] 1 AC 310, 418. See also *ibid*, 401, *per* Lord Ackner.

(5)   Where the defendant has negligently damaged or imperilled property belonging to the plaintiff or a third party, and the plaintiff, as a result, has foreseeably suffered a psychiatric illness, it would appear that, in certain circumstances, the plaintiff can recover for that illness but the necessary criteria for recovery are unclear.

2.42   In *Owens v Liverpool Corporation*[131] relatives of a deceased person, whose coffin was overturned when the defendant's tram driver negligently collided with the hearse, recovered damages for "nervous shock". The Court of Appeal held that the right to recover damages for psychiatric illness caused by the negligence of a defendant was not limited to cases in which apprehension as to human safety was involved. MacKinnon LJ, delivering the judgment of the court, thought that damages might even be recoverable where the plaintiff's illness was caused by shock from apprehension as to the life of a beloved pet such as a dog.[132]

2.43   Although doubt was cast on the decision in *Owens v Liverpool Corporation* in *Bourhill v Young*[133] and by Lord Oliver in *Alcock*,[134] recovery for shock-induced psychiatric illness suffered as a result of either apprehended or actual harm to property was not expressly ruled out in either case. Most importantly, in *Attia v British Gas Plc*[135] it was accepted on a preliminary issue that a claim for damages in respect of shock arising out of damage to property (the destruction by fire of the plaintiff's home) could in principle succeed, and the matter was allowed to proceed to trial. The Court of Appeal refused to accept the argument that there was any rule of policy excluding liability for shock-induced psychiatric illness caused by witnessing damage to one's property. Bingham LJ said, "Suppose, for example, that a scholar's life's work of research or composition were destroyed before his eyes as a result of a defendant's careless conduct, causing the scholar to suffer reasonably foreseeable psychiatric damage. Or suppose that a householder returned home to find that his most cherished possessions had been destroyed through the carelessness of an intruder in starting a fire or leaving a tap running, causing reasonably foreseeable psychiatric damage to the owner. I do not think a legal principle which forbade recovery in these circumstances could be supported."[136] The Court of Appeal did not, of course, attempt to lay down all the criteria which should be applied by a court when determining whether damages for shock-induced psychiatric illness are

---

[131]   [1939] 1 KB 394.

[132]   *Ibid*, 399.

[133]   [1943] AC 92, 100, 110, 116. Lord Thankerton had difficulty in seeing that there was any relationship of duty between the parties on the facts. Lord Wright, on the other hand, thought that the particular susceptibility in *Owens* was beyond any range of normal expectancy or of reasonable foresight. Lord Porter disagreed with the Court of Appeal's decision on both grounds.

[134]   [1992] 1 AC 310, 412.

[135]   [1988] QB 304.

[136]   *Ibid*, 320.

recoverable in cases like these. For example, would the plaintiff have succeeded in her claim if the house had belonged to, say, her husband? And does the value, or kind, of property matter?[137]

2.44   Where property *belonging to the plaintiff* has been damaged, one can argue that consequent psychiatric illness should be recoverable without special restrictions in the same way that psychiatric illness consequent on a physical injury to the plaintiff is recoverable without special restrictions. It may also be significant that in that situation the plaintiff is a primary and not a secondary victim. That no special restrictions apply in that situation is supported by dicta in *Attia v British Gas Plc*,[138] although the facts of that case were "strong" in that the plaintiff had witnessed the property damage occurring and her psychiatric illness was shock-induced. On the other hand, it may be argued that it would be odd if a plaintiff could recover more easily for psychiatric illness consequent on damage to his or her property (for example, a house) than for psychiatric illness consequent on personal injury to another (for example, his or her spouse). Certainly where the property damaged or imperilled *belongs to a third party*, one would expect that criteria should be satisfied that are analogous to, but no less restrictive than, those applied where another person's safety is involved. For example, it is presumably necessary that the plaintiff has a "close relationship" to the property (for instance, by living in a house, albeit not one's own); that the psychiatric illness was suffered from being present around the time when the damage occurred and from perceiving the damage rather than being told of it; and that the psychiatric illness was shock-induced.

(6) It is unclear whether there can be liability for the negligent communication of news to the plaintiff which has foreseeably caused him or her to suffer a psychiatric illness.

2.45   May a person be liable in the tort of negligence for communicating false news, or true news in an insensitive style, thereby causing the plaintiff a foreseeable psychiatric illness?[139] If the news concerns someone other than the plaintiff (for example, that a loved one has been killed or injured) the *Alcock* requirement of direct sensory perception of the accident would necessarily bar all claims against the

---

[137] N J Mullany and P R Handford, *Tort Liability for Psychiatric Damage* (1993) pp 211-212.

[138] [1988] QB 304, 312, *per* Dillon LJ; 317, *per* Woolf LJ. See also *Campbelltown City Council v Mackay* (1989) 15 NSWLR 501 in which the plaintiffs were awarded damages in the tort of negligence for psychiatric illness, as part of their damages for vexation and inconvenience, when their new house cracked and ultimately had to be demolished: this was so even though the psychiatric illness was gradually sustained and not shock-induced. For discussion, see N J Mullany and P R Handford, *Tort Liability for Psychiatric Damage* (1993) pp 201-202.

[139] We do not here discuss psychiatric illness caused to a plaintiff by statements about the plaintiff made to a third party. In general, liability in that situation will lie, if at all, in the tort of defamation, not in the tort of negligence. Nor do we here discuss *M v Newham LBC* [1994] 2 WLR 554 in which the plaintiffs' alleged psychiatric illness followed from the action of a third party relying on the false statements of the defendant: see para 2.6 above.

conveyers of news. But that requirement was formulated in respect of claims by secondary victims against the person responsible for the accident itself and was presumably not intended to rule out claims for negligent communication. Indeed, in relation to the negligent communication, rather than the negligence causing the accident, the plaintiff is perhaps more aptly regarded as a primary, rather than a secondary, victim. And the *Alcock* requirement is obviously inappropriate where the bad news relates to the plaintiff rather than a third party, as where a person is bluntly given the news that she has a terminal illness in a hospital corridor.

2.46 There is no English authority directly in point on the question whether those communicating bad news which is *true* have a duty to communicate it carefully.[140] In Australia Windeyer J has said that "[i]f the sole cause of shock be what is told or read of some happening then I think it is correctly said that, unless there be an intention to cause a nervous shock, no action lies against ... the bearer of the bad tidings .... There is no duty in law to break bad news gently ...."[141] And in the Court of Appeal in *Alcock*, Parker LJ thought that a person informing a parent of a child's death or multiple injuries "cannot be held liable for obvious reasons".[142] However, in *Winfield and Jolowicz on Tort* it is suggested that where the impact of the news is needlessly exacerbated liability may well be imposed.[143]

2.47 There is similarly no English authority concerning liability for psychiatric illness caused by the negligent communication of bad news which is *false* - for example, where a newspaper negligently reports the false news that one's husband has been seriously injured or where the police wrongly inform a mother of her child's death.

---

[140] In the context of statements made by employers in job references which cause the employee *economic* loss, Lord Woolf has said that there can be no action for negligence if the statement is true: *Spring v Guardian Assurance Plc* [1994] 3 WLR 354, 398. A recent case, mentioned in the *Daily Telegraph* of 1 February 1995, concerned claims for psychiatric illness by women who were told by letter that they had been treated by a health worker with HIV. We understand that it was admitted by the defendant health authorities that there was a duty of care not to break the news in an insensitive way; and that no authorities on the point were cited to, or referred to by, French J.

[141] *Mount Isa Mines Ltd v Pusey* (1970) 125 CLR 383, 407 (High Court of Australia).

[142] [1992] 1 AC 310, 363. It was unnecessary for the Court of Appeal or the House of Lords in *Alcock* to address the question whether, if there had been a breach of the broadcasting code of ethics, the television authorities could themselves have been liable for the shock-induced psychiatric illness caused to the plaintiffs.

[143] (14th ed 1994) p 124. Similarly, it is Professor Walker's view that liability might be imposed upon the person communicating true bad news if he or she did not take reasonable care to break it as gently as possible, eg where a policeman tells a woman of her husband's death in the phrase, "Mrs X, your man's dead.": D M Walker, *The Law of Delict in Scotland* (2nd ed 1981) p 678, n 77. In the South Australian case of *Brown v Mount Barker Soldiers' Hospital Inc* [1934] SASR 128 the plaintiff recovered for the shock which she suffered on being informed by the hospital authorities in whose care she was that her baby had been injured as a result of their negligence (nb: a duty of care was owed to the plaintiff as a hospital in-patient). See also the New Zealand case, *Furniss v Fitchett* [1958] NZLR 396 in which the plaintiff recovered damages from her doctor for psychiatric illness caused by his negligent disclosure of his opinion as to her mental stability.

Tortious liability exists for false statements causing psychiatric illness which are made knowingly and intentionally under *Wilkinson v Downton*,[144] but Lord Denning MR has expressed the view, *obiter*, that it would be "a big step forward - or backward" to extend that authority to false statements made honestly and in good faith.[145] However, it is well established that a duty of care exists in respect of negligent misstatements which give rise to *physical* injury[146] and even that, in special circumstances, false statements which give rise to purely economic loss are actionable in negligence.[147] Analogies with other areas of tort law also indicate that the courts might be more inclined to recognise a duty of care in respect of false statements than in respect of those which are true.[148]

2.48   In the Canadian case of *Guay v Sun Publishing Co*[149] a newspaper had carelessly published a false news item that the plaintiff's husband and three children had been killed in a motor accident. The plaintiff read the item and allegedly suffered shock-induced psychiatric illness. A majority of the Supreme Court of Canada held that the plaintiff's claim in negligence against the newspaper should be dismissed, but differed in their reasons.[150] The dissenting judges took the view that there was no reason why the plaintiff's claim should not succeed.[151] The decision in *Guay* was made at a time when liability for negligent statements - whatever the nature of the injury caused - was questionable, and it has been argued that "[i]n the light of subsequent developments ... one might safely forecast that the Supreme Court of Canada would impose liability on similar facts today."[152] And it should be noted

---

[144] [1897] 2 QB 57. See para 1.4 above.

[145] *D v NSPCC* [1978] AC 171, 188-189. He posed the example of a person who has a nervous breakdown through shock on being informed by a policeman that he is suspected, wrongly, of being a thief.

[146] Eg *Clayton v Woodman & Son (Builders) Ltd* [1962] 2 QB 533.

[147] The leading authority is *Hedley Byrne & Co Ltd v Heller & Partners Ltd* [1964] AC 465.

[148] Eg it would seem that damages for psychiatric illness caused by false statements may be recovered as part of an action for defamation: see para 1.5 n 17 above.

[149] [1953] 4 DLR 577 (S Ct of Canada).

[150] Locke J was of the view that there could be no liability at all for negligent statements, whatever the nature of the harm caused; Kerwin J held that on the facts, no duty of care was owed because injury to the plaintiff was not reasonably foreseeable; whilst Estey J thought that there was a lack of evidence that the plaintiff had suffered psychiatric illness as a result of reading the news and refused to decide whether there could ever be liability for nervous shock resulting from negligent misstatements.

[151] Cartwright J and Rinfret CJC.

[152] A M Linden, *Canadian Tort Law* (4th ed 1988) p 397, who notes that in 1973 the Ontario CA reversed without reasons a trial decision which relied on *Guay*: see *Hurley v Sault Star* (unreported, 16 November 1973).

that in Australia damages have been awarded for psychiatric illness caused by the negligent communication of false information.[153]

(7) There are miscellaneous instances (ie other than those covered by propositions (3) (5) and (6) above) where a primary victim probably can recover for a psychiatric illness foreseeably caused by the defendant's negligence.

2.49 The most important decision here is *Walker v Northumberland CC*,[154] in which Colman J held that a social worker, dealing with a high number of child abuse cases, was entitled to damages from his employer in the tort of negligence (and in contract) for a second nervous breakdown caused by stress at work. Colman J said, "It is clear law that an employer has a duty to provide his employee with a reasonably safe system of work and to take reasonable steps to protect him from risks which are reasonably foreseeable. Whereas the law on the extent of this duty has developed almost exclusively in cases involving physical injury to the employee as distinct from injury to his mental health, there is no logical reason why risk of psychiatric damage should be excluded from the scope of an employer's duty of care or from the co-extensive implied term in the contract of employment."[155] The judge went on to emphasise that, as regards psychiatric illness, the application of the law will often give rise to factual difficulties, given that professional work is intrinsically demanding and stressful. On the facts, he thought that the defendants were not in breach of their duty of care as regards the plaintiff's first nervous breakdown because it was not then reasonably foreseeable that the work-load to which the plaintiff was exposed gave rise to a material risk of mental illness. However, when the plaintiff returned to work the defendants, knowing of his previous breakdown, ought to have taken steps, as the plaintiff had been led to believe they would, to alleviate his excessive work-load. They were therefore in breach of their duty of care as regards his second nervous breakdown.

2.50 This is a landmark decision and, if upheld on appeal, it is likely to lead to other successful claims by employees against their employers for psychiatric illness suffered through work. It is noteworthy that Mr Walker's psychiatric illness was not shock-induced. That Colman J did not consider it necessary even to refer to *Alcock*,

---

[153] *Barnes v Commonwealth of Australia* (1937) 37 SR (NSW) 511: see Appendix, para 8 n 29 below. See generally, N J Mullany and P R Handford, *Tort Liability for Psychiatric Illness* (1993) pp 183-191.

[154] (1994) 144 NLJ 1659; noted B McKenna, "Stress injuries at work" (1994) 144 NLJ 1652. See also *Gillespie v Commonwealth of Australia* (1991) 104 ACTR 1: see Appendix, para 13 below. A similar claim failed on the facts in *Petch v Customs and Excise Commissioners* [1993] ICR 789 (CA). See further *Johnstone v Bloomsbury Health Authority* [1992] QB 333 in which the Court of Appeal (Leggatt LJ dissenting) refused an application to strike out a doctor's claim for stress and depression brought about by long working hours albeit that a term of his contract obliged him to be available for up to 48 hours on average per week overtime, in addition to the basic working week of 40 hours.

[155] (1994) 144 NLJ 1659.

nor any other "nervous shock" case, supports the view, discussed above,[156] that in a primary victim case like this, as opposed to a secondary victim case like *Alcock*, it is not a pre-requisite for liability that the psychiatric illness has been shock-induced.

2.51 Other miscellaneous situations in which a primary victim *probably* can recover for a negligently inflicted psychiatric illness (assuming the standard elements of the tort of negligence can be made out) include: where a patient suffers a psychiatric illness because of negligent treatment by his psychiatrist;[157] where a stage hypnotist causes an unsuspecting volunteer foreseeably to suffer a psychiatric illness following hypnosis;[158] and where a prisoner foreseeably suffers a psychiatric illness as a result of ill-treatment by prison officers.[159]

PRINCIPLES OF ASSESSMENT AND LEVELS OF DAMAGES

2.52 Although this paper is concerned with matters of liability rather than the assessment of damages, a brief exposition of how damages for psychiatric illness are assessed may be of help in enabling one to appreciate the full range of issues confronting the law.

2.53 The principles upon which damages for psychiatric illness are assessed are the same as those which apply in the case of any other personal injury.[160] Thus, on the principle that the plaintiff is to be put into the position he or she would have been in had the wrong not occurred,[161] damages will be awarded to cover both the plaintiff's pecuniary loss (such as the cost of psychiatric treatment and loss of earnings if ability to work is impaired) and non-pecuniary loss (that is, for any pain, suffering and loss of amenity).[162] However, although in principle it is the same, the assessment of damages for psychiatric illness is in some respects more difficult and imprecise than that for physical injury, and it has been said that damages are more than usually at large.[163] First, although all assessments of damages in cases of serious personal injury involve an element of uncertainty and speculation, this is especially

---

[156] See paras 2.6-2.7 above.

[157] Cf *M v Newham LBC* [1994] 2 WLR 554: see paragraph 2.6 above.

[158] This type of case has recently been discussed in the media: see, eg, *The Times* 14 December 1994, p 8.

[159] Cf *R v Deputy Governor of Parkhurst Prison, ex p Hague* [1992] 1 AC 58, 165-166, *per* Lord Bridge; *Racz v Home Office* [1994] 2 AC 45 (but note that in that case mental distress alone had been suffered and the central cause of action was misfeasance in public office, not negligence).

[160] See, generally, *Kemp and Kemp*, vol 1, ch 1; vol 2, paras C4-001 and C4-002.

[161] This is the basic compensatory aim, stated by Lord Blackburn in *Livingstone v Rawyards Coal Co* (1880) 5 App Cas 25, 39.

[162] Eg feelings of insecurity and fear, inability to participate fully in the normal activities of life, loss of sexual function.

[163] *Hinz v Berry* [1970] 2 QB 40, 46, *per* Sir Gordon Willmer.

so where psychiatric illness is concerned.[164] For instance, there is much room for difference of opinion between medical experts as to the gravity of the plaintiff's psychiatric illness and his or her prognosis.[165] Secondly, the precise effects and nature of psychiatric illness vary widely from individual to individual, even where the same type of disorder (or diagnosis) is involved. Thirdly, psychiatric illness is often medically attributable to a whole range of factors which may be difficult to separate out,[166] yet for the purposes of the law it is only shock-induced psychiatric damage which is actionable (at least in the case of secondary victims) and hence for which damages may be recovered.[167]

2.54   As regards non-pecuniary loss, the Judicial Studies Board's *Guidelines for the Assessment of General Damages in Personal Injury Cases*[168] indicate a possible range of from £500 for very minor psychiatric illness to £45,000 for very severe psychiatric illness[169] and further suggest that the factors which will be relevant to the precise level of the award in any particular case may include the following: ability to cope with life and particularly work, effect on relationships with family etc, extent to which treatment would be successful, future vulnerability, future prognosis and whether medical help has been sought. It may be that the range of awards for psychiatric illness will become more specific in the future, corresponding to specific types of the most common disorders.[170] The *Guidelines*, for instance, now include a separate category for post-traumatic stress disorder.

---

[164] *Kemp and Kemp*, vol 2, para C4-002.

[165] Eg *Tuckey v R & H Green and Silley Weir Ltd* [1955] 2 Lloyd's Rep 619, 630. In contrast, the permanency of physical injury, such as the loss of a limb, is usually clear and unproblematic.

[166] Disregarding the special case of disease, physical injury is usually caused by a single event or accident (impact) attributable to the defendant's negligence. In addition, pre-existing susceptibility is more relevant to psychiatric than to physical injury.

[167] See para 2.8 above.

[168] (2nd ed 1994) p 10.

[169] The rough maximum of £45,000 for psychiatric damage compares with the unofficial maximum of £125,000 for the most severe type of physical injury (quadriplegia). In *R v Liverpool City Council*, 23 November 1988, *Kemp and Kemp*, vol 2, para C4-022, Hodgson J described the levels of damages for psychiatric injury in comparison with those for physical injuries as "surprisingly low". In *Hale v London Underground Ltd* [1993] PIQR Q30 a fireman who suffered psychiatric damage but no physical injury in the King's Cross fire was awarded damages totalling £144,390, including £27,500 for non-pecuniary loss. In *Vernon v Bosley* (unreported, 30 January 1995) a father who, twelve years before trial, had witnessed the immediate aftermath of the drowning of his two daughters, and was held to have suffered features of both post-traumatic stress disorder and pathological grief, was awarded £1,178,527, of which only £37,500 was for non-pecuniary loss.

[170] N J Mullany and P R Handford, *Tort Liability for Psychiatric Damage* (1993) ch 13, suggest that a tariff for non-pecuniary loss might be organised according to specific types of psychiatric disorder.

2.55 We shall be examining the assessment of damages for non-pecuniary loss in personal injury cases generally in a forthcoming consultation paper.[171] Nevertheless **we would welcome the views of consultees now on the following question: are the problems of assessing damages for psychiatric illness thought to be so much greater than for other types of personal injury, that a different method or regime should be adopted for the assessment of damages for psychiatric illness than is adopted for assessing damages for other types of personal injury?**

---

[171] See para 1.1 n 3 above.

PART III
THE MEDICAL BACKGROUND

3.1 The law in the area of negligently inflicted psychiatric illness has been influenced by medical opinion. It clearly cannot be right to discuss the law's possible future development without some awareness of current medical thinking. Indeed it can be argued that any rational restatement of the law on psychiatric illness must start from the medical understanding of such illness. With this in mind, we attempt in this Part to give a brief overview of some of the relevant medical literature and studies.[1] In doing so, we have not attempted a survey of all the psychiatric illnesses that could conceivably be compensatable in a negligence action. Instead we have focused on shock-induced psychiatric illnesses, and especially post-traumatic stress disorder.

(1) Shock-induced psychiatric illness

3.2 Medical opinion has changed considerably in the last half century. In earlier years the consensus among psychiatrists was that lasting damage did not occur in "normal" individuals as a result of emotional shock, however severe the shock.[2] It is now acknowledged, however, that a shock may be sufficient to produce a psychiatric illness on its own.[3]

3.3 The psychiatric profession now has two diagnostic classificatory systems.[4] These are the American Diagnostic and Statistical Manual of Mental Disorders (DSM-IV)[5] and the International Classification of Diseases and Related Health Problems (ICD-10).[6] The first edition of the Diagnostic and Statistical Manual of Mental Disorders, DSM-I, was published by the American Psychiatric Association in 1952. DSM-IV was published in 1994, succeeding a revised third edition which was published in 1987 and known as DSM-III-R. The International Classification of Diseases and Related Health Problems, meanwhile, is published by the World Health Organisation. The first edition to include psychiatric illnesses was the sixth, which was published in the 1950s. Subsequent editions developed the classifications

---

[1] See para 2.4 above for some of the main types of recognised psychiatric illness that have qualified for compensation. For another survey of the medical background, see N J Mullany and P R Handford, *op cit*, pp 24-42. See also Deane J's review of propositions gained from expert opinion in *Jaensch v Coffey* (1984) 155 CLR 549, 600-601.

[2] See P Milici (1939) 13 Psychiatric Quarterly 278 and D Palmer (1954) 1 Journal of Forensic Medicine 225 considered in J Havard, "Reasonable Foresight of Nervous Shock" (1956) 19 MLR 478, 482. See also H W Smith, "Relation of Emotions to Injury and Disease: Legal Liability for Psychic Stimuli" (1944) 30 Va LR 193, esp 225, 302.

[3] See para 3.5 below.

[4] M Gelder, D Gath and R Mayou, *Oxford Textbook of Psychiatry* (2nd ed 1988) pp 87-91; D Healy, *Images of Trauma* (1993) pp 78-79. These classificatory systems are also used by psychologists.

[5] 4th Edition, 1994 (DSM-IV): American Psychiatric Association.

[6] Tenth Revision, Volume 1, 1993 (ICD-10): World Health Organisation.

further, particularly ICD-8, published in 1965, and ICD-10, which was published in 1993.

3.4 A plaintiff may suffer more than one psychiatric illness following trauma[7] and, indeed, studies indicate that this frequently occurs.[8] A plaintiff cannot usually point to organic or physical symptoms as proof that he or she has a psychiatric illness. There may often only be intangible symptoms of which the patient complains, and behavioural manifestations which are apparent to observers.[9] Since the identification and assessment of symptoms is often based on the complainant's own report, there may be suspicions of malingering and disagreement as to the extent of injury in some cases.[10] In cases of psychiatric illness causation is generally inferred only on the basis of common occurrence,[11] timing, and (possibly) by means of a link between the type of trauma that has occurred and specific personal vulnerability.[12] It should be noted that DSM-IV specifically states that it was developed for clinical, educational and research purposes and cautions that in most cases the clinical diagnosis of a DSM-IV mental disorder will not in itself suffice to establish the existence of a mental disorder for legal purposes, owing to the imperfect fit between

[7] DSM-IV, para 309.81, p 427 states that a diagnosis of Brief Psychotic Disorder, Conversion Disorder or Major Depressive Disorder may be given in addition to Posttraumatic Stress Disorder. There is also an increased risk of Panic Disorder, Agoraphobia, Obsessive-Compulsive Disorder, Social Phobia, Specific Phobia, Somatization Disorder, Major Depressive Disorder and Substance-Related Disorders where Posttraumatic Stress Disorder is diagnosed: para 309.81, p 425.

[8] E Brett, "Classifications of Posttraumatic Stress Disorder in DSM-IV: Anxiety Disorder, Dissociative Disorder, or Stress Disorder?" in J Davidson and E Foa (eds), *Posttraumatic Stress Disorder: DSM-IV and Beyond* (1993) p 191 at p 193 (PTSD co-occurs most frequently with substance abuse, depression, and anxiety disorders). In a study of firefighters exposed to a natural disaster, McFarlane and Papay found that only 23% of the 70 subjects who had developed PTSD did not attract a further diagnosis, with major depression being the most common concurrent disorder: A McFarlane and P Papay, "Multiple Diagnoses in Posttraumatic Stress Disorder in the Victims of a Natural Disaster" (1992) 180 Journal of Nervous and Mental Disease 498, 502.

[9] M Weller, "Compensation for psychiatric disability" in R Bluglass and P Bowden (eds), *Principles and Practice of Forensic Psychiatry* (1990) p 1101 at p 1102.

[10] See D Enoch, "Hysteria, malingering, pseudologica fantastica, Ganser syndrome, prison psychosis and Münchausen's syndrome" in R Bluglass and P Bowden (eds), *Principles and Practice of Forensic Psychiatry* (1990) p 805 at pp 805-811; L J Raifman, "Problems of Diagnosis and Legal Causation in Courtroom Use of Post-Traumatic Stress Disorder" (1983) 1 Behavioral Sciences and the Law 115, 121 and 124. See paras 4.7-4.9 below.

[11] M Gelder, D Gath and R Mayou, *Oxford Textbook of Psychiatry* (2nd ed 1988) pp 95-98; M Weller, "Compensation for psychiatric disability" in R Bluglass and P Bowden (eds), *Principles and Practice of Forensic Psychiatry* (1990) p 1103 at p 1105; H W Smith, "Relation of Emotions to Injury and Disease: Legal Liability for Psychic Stimuli" (1943) 30 Va LR 193, 215.

[12] N Eastman, "Psychiatric Negligence and Psychological Damages" in "Shock, Pain and Trauma: Psychiatric Aspects of Civil Litigation" (MIND conference, February 1993) p 8. On the controversy about predisposing vulnerability, see para 3.9 below.

the questions that are of ultimate concern to the law and the information that is contained in a clinical diagnosis.[13]

(2) Post-traumatic stress disorder (PTSD)

3.5   A significant proportion of the plaintiffs who have claimed damages for psychiatric illness in the past decade have formulated their claims specifically in terms of post-traumatic stress disorder (PTSD). This concept of PTSD has crystallised in psychiatric diagnostic classification at a time when the public and the courts have been particularly receptive to such a phenomenon, possibly because of disasters such as those that took place at Hillsborough and Zeebrugge.[14] Although there may be cases in which awards of compensation for damages caused by the defendant's negligence are made for shock-induced psychiatric illness other than PTSD,[15] PTSD is the most common diagnosis where shock is the initiating factor, and "the reality is that borderline cases of nervous shock are influenced by psychiatric criteria for PTSD."[16] The increasing prominence of PTSD in personal injury claims is also attributable in part to a lessening in the resistance to the concept of trauma and mental disorder in the behavioural sciences.[17] PTSD was first introduced as a

---

[13]   DSM-IV, Introduction, p xxiii and Cautionary Statement, p xxvii. See also B Hoffman and H Spiegel, "Legal Principles in the Psychiatric Assessment of Personal Injury Litigants" (1989) 146 American Journal of Psychiatry 304, esp 309.

[14]   See M Weller, "Post traumatic stress disorder" (1993) 143 NLJ 878; C Pugh and M Trimble, "Psychiatric Injury After Hillsborough" (1993) 163 British Journal of Psychiatry 425; N J Mullany and P R Handford, *op cit*, p 34 nn 101-102. On the response of the criminal courts, see R Rosser, S Dewar and J Thompson, "Psychological aftermath of the King's Cross fire" (1991) 84 Journal of the Royal Society of Medicine 4, 7. Other recent disasters which have contributed to this process include the Piper Alpha oil rig disaster and the Marchioness riverboat disaster.

[15]   See para 2.4 above. Responses to trauma may be a variety of stress response syndromes, including, but not limited to, PTSD: B Green, "Defining Trauma: Terminology and Generic Stressor Dimensions" (1990) 20 Journal of Applied Social Psychology 1632, 1639. Davidson and Foa point to the growing recognition that, in all probability, other forms of abnormal post-traumatic stress reactions exist in addition to PTSD, and that in fact there are eight such disorders referred to in the relevant literature including brief reactive psychosis, dream anxiety disorders, conversion and somatization disorders, multiple personality disorder, and some types of borderline personality disorder: J Davidson and E Foa, Epilogue to J Davidson and E Foa (eds), *Posttraumatic Stress Disorder: DSM-IV and Beyond* (1993) p 229 at p 234. Green warns against over-dependence on the criteria for post-traumatic stress disorder for defining stressors and responses, and states that there are other types of experiences, or lower intensity experiences, which may have chronic psychological effects that are not PTSD: B Green, *op cit*, 1639.

[16]   R English, "Nervous Shock: Before the Aftermath" [1993] CLJ 204, 205.

[17]   See para 4.5 below. Since the beginning of psychiatry there has been a controversy on the question whether traumatic events could lead to lasting psychopathology. This was very evident in the first two versions of the diagnostic and statistical manual of the American Psychiatric Association, published in 1952 and 1968. In DSM-I(I), for example, trauma could only lead to "gross stress reactions" which were part of "transient situational personality disorders". Extreme stress events were thought to lead only to a transient or temporary disturbance, and if symptoms were more severe, a different diagnosis had to be made: see D Brom, R Kleber and E Witztum, "The Prevalence of Posttraumatic Psychopathology in the General and the Clinical Population" (1992) 28 Israel Journal of

psychiatric diagnostic category in the American Diagnostic and Statistical Manual of Mental Disorders in 1980[18] and is now represented in both the fourth edition of this manual, DSM-IV,[19] and also in the International Classification of Diseases, ICD-10.[20] The main feature of the disorder is the development of characteristic symptoms following a psychologically distressing event or situation of an exceptionally threatening or catastrophic nature.[21] In DSM-III-R it was specified that the event or situation in question must have been outside the range of usual human experience, and this 1987 revised manual contained a list of stressors[22] which would not qualify. These included "such common experiences as simple bereavement, chronic illness, business losses, and marital conflict".[23] Both DSM-III-R and ICD-10 specified that the event must be such as would be likely to cause marked or pervasive distress to almost anyone.[24] DSM-IV requires the stressor to have been "extreme" and it goes on to list two characteristics of the initiating event which must have been present for a diagnosis of PTSD to be made. These are: (1) that the person in question experienced, witnessed, or was confronted with an event or events that involved actual or threatened death or serious injury, or a threat to the physical integrity of self or others, and (2) that his or her response involved intense fear, helplessness, or horror.[25] Significantly, the stressor may consist of

Psychiatry & Related Sciences 53.

[18] DSM-III, 1980, p 237, revised in 1987. However, it is acknowledged that this was far from being the first recognition of psychiatric symptoms following traumatic events and that the condition has in fact been around for many years albeit under a different nomenclature, for example, "traumatic neurosis" and "shell shock". See B Gersons and I Carlier, "Post-traumatic Stress Disorder: The History of a Recent Concept" (1992) 161 British Journal of Psychiatry 742; M Trimble, *Post-Traumatic Neurosis: From Railway Spine to the Whiplash* (1981). PTSD was included in DSM-III as a compromise after veterans' groups and mental health personnel engaged in caring for Vietnam veterans spearheaded a drive for the recognition of a "post-Vietnam syndrome": J Helzer, L Robins and L McEvoy, "Post-Traumatic Stress Disorder in the General Population" (1987) 317 New England Journal of Medicine 1630.

[19] DSM-IV, para 309.81, p 424.

[20] ICD-10, 1993, para F43.1, p 344.

[21] ICD-10, para F43.1, p 344. Where significant psychiatric symptoms follow stressors of a more "ordinary" kind, this is considered a maladaptation to be diagnosed as adjustment disorder, an acute syndrome designed to cover overreactions (by vulnerable persons) to life difficulties: N Breslau and G Davis, "Posttraumatic Stress Disorder: The Stressor Criterion" (1987) 175 Journal of Nervous and Mental Disease 255, 260.

[22] An event or change that may be temporally (and perhaps causally) connected with the onset, occurrence, or exacerbation of a mental disorder.

[23] DSM-III-R, para 309.89, p 247.

[24] ICD-10, para F43.1, p 344; DSM-III-R, para 309.89, p 247.

[25] DSM-IV, para 309.81, p 424.

merely *learning about* unexpected or violent death, serious harm, or threat of death or injury experienced by a family member or other close associate.[26]

3.6 PTSD is unique in psychiatric classification in that it contains an explicit assumption that the cause of the disorder is known.[27] Since the diagnosis cannot be made unless there has been an exposure to an external causative event, and since in both diagnostic classificatory systems it is assumed, in the formulation of PTSD, that the sufferer's symptoms are a consequence of the exposure to this event,[28] it is hardly surprising that it has been suggested that, in cases where a diagnosis of PTSD is accepted, a plaintiff's action for damages for PTSD is most unlikely to fail on the issue of causation.[29] Although a diagnosis of PTSD will not be excluded where there are also "internal factors" in existence - such as personality traits which predispose the sufferer to psychiatric illness - the prevailing view today is that the existence of such factors are neither necessary nor sufficient themselves to explain the occurrence of PTSD.[30] Other psychiatric diagnoses - such as anxiety, neurosis or depression - do not depend upon the identification of the precipitating factors, and personal weakness or vulnerability plays a much more important role. In such cases, therefore, the causal link between the psychiatric condition and the defendant's negligence is far more difficult to demonstrate.

[26] DSM-IV, para 309.81, p 424. However, not everyone develops PTSD even in reaction to an extremely serious stressor and the traumatic stressful event is insufficient in itself to warrant a diagnosis of PTSD: see generally, B Gersons and I Carlier, "Post-traumatic Stress Disorder: The History of a Recent Concept" (1992) 161 British Journal of Psychiatry 742. See paras 3.10-3.15 below on prevalence and statistical probability.

[27] See M Weller, "Post traumatic stress disorder" (1993) 143 NLJ 878; D Healy, *Images of Trauma* (1993) pp 104-106. Characteristic symptoms of PTSD include (1) persistent re-experiencing of the traumatic event, (2) persistent avoidance of stimuli associated with the trauma and "psychic numbing" and (3) persistent symptoms of anxiety or increased arousal: DSM-IV, para 309.81, p 424. ICD-10 lists characteristic symptoms similar to those specified in DSM-III-R, but in contrast it does not require that the sufferer should have displayed any particular number of these before a diagnosis of PTSD may be made.

[28] See ICD-10, para F43.1, p 344 and DSM-IV, para 309.81, p 424. An additional requirement of DSM-IV is that disturbance, namely the listed symptoms, must last for at least one month before a diagnosis of PTSD can be made: para 309.81, p 424. When the duration of symptoms is less than three months, PTSD should be specified as "acute". If symptoms last beyond that period, PTSD should be specified as "chronic": DSM-IV, para 309.81, p 425. DSM-IV also requires that the disturbance should have caused clinically significant distress or impairment in social, occupational, or other important areas of functioning before a diagnosis can be made: para 309.81, p 424.

[29] G Mezey, "Assessing Emotional and Psychological Harm: 'Post Traumatic Stress Disorder'" in "Shock, Pain and Trauma: Psychiatric Aspects of Civil Litigation" (MIND conference, February 1993) pp 6-7; letter by M Weller (1993) 143 NLJ 1186. An obvious exception to this would be where the plaintiff has been exposed to several shocking events (eg a fireman working at several disasters) only one of which was caused by another's negligence.

[30] ICD-10, para F43.1, p 344. See also para 3.9 below.

3.7 Both DSM-IV[31] and the diagnostic guidelines in ICD-10[32] provide examples of events that fall within the criteria they set out. The list in DSM-IV, however, is more comprehensive and it distinguishes between traumatic events which are directly experienced, those which are witnessed and those which are learnt about. Examples of the first include natural or man-made disasters, severe automobile accidents, or the shock of being diagnosed with a life-threatening illness.[33] Examples of the second might include the experience of seeing someone being seriously injured or killed in an accident, seeing a violent assault, war, or other disaster, or the experience of unexpectedly witnessing a dead body or parts of a body. Examples of the third category might include the experience of learning about a violent personal assault, a serious accident, or a serious injury to a member of one's family or a close friend; or learning about the sudden, unexpected death of such a person; or learning that one's child has a life-threatening disease.[34] In DSM-IV it is said that the disorder may be particularly severe or long-lasting when the stressor is of human design.[35]

3.8 Reviews of the empirical studies in the psychiatric and legal literature that are concerned with traumatic stress reactions affirm that threat to life and physical well-being - either to oneself or to a loved one - severe physical injury, exposure to grotesque death, witnessing death, and hearing about death are major risk factors

---

[31] DSM-IV, para 309.81, p 424.

[32] ICD-10 Classification of Mental and Behavioural Disorders: Clinical descriptions and diagnostic guidelines (1992) para F43.1, p 147.

[33] Other listed stressors which the sufferer might have directly experienced, but which are less significant for our purposes, include military combat, violent personal assault, the experience of being kidnapped or taken hostage, terrorist attack, and incarceration as a prisoner of war: DSM-IV, para 309.81, p 424. See also ICD-10 Classification of Mental and Behavioural Disorders: Clinical descriptions and diagnostic guidelines (1992) para F43.1, p 147.

[34] DSM-IV, para 309.81, p 424. The examples given are wider than those given in the ICD-10 Classification of Mental and Behavioural Disorders: Clinical descriptions and diagnostic guidelines (1992) para F43.1, p 147. Whilst ordinary bereavement will not suffice for a diagnosis of PTSD, where the loss of a loved one is caused by a violent traumatic event, although the stressor would be the experience of hearing about the death, the person concerned would be likely to perceive the event vicariously. This has been documented as a form of exposure to an event that can predict PTSD symptoms: B Green, "Defining Trauma: Terminology and Generic Stressor Dimensions" (1990) 20 Journal of Applied Social Psychology 1632, 1637. Lundin, for example, found an especially high increase in psychiatric illness after sudden and unexpected bereavement, possibly attributable to the unexpectedness of the deaths: T Lundin, "Morbidity following Sudden and Unexpected Bereavement" (1984) 144 British Journal of Psychiatry 84, 87. However, Lundin's study was not confined to bereavement as a result of accident, but included loss due to disease. Moreover, he did not differentiate between different psychiatric diagnoses in the survivors.

[35] DSM-IV, para 309.81, p 424. For consideration of the types of trauma, see C B Scrignar, *Post-Traumatic Stress Disorder: Disorder, Treatment, and Legal Issues* (2nd ed 1988) pp 42-61.

for the development of PTSD.[36] In addition, both the current diagnostic systems (ICD-10 and DSM-IV) implicitly acknowledge the importance of subjective perception whilst continuing to define PTSD as a trauma-driven disorder.[37] Aspects of subjective perception which are common to PTSD-sufferers and are documented in the empirical material include the perception of threat to life, the perceived potential for physical violence, the experience of extreme fear, and the attribution of personal helplessness.[38]

3.9　Some commentators maintain that a predisposition to psychiatric illness is an important factor in the development of PTSD however extreme the external event may be.[39] However, the more commonly accepted view today is that, while in a case of a trauma of less extreme severity the development of PTSD will depend on both external and internal factors, certain extreme types of traumatic event are likely to induce PTSD (at least initially) in most people regardless of predisposition.[40] It is

[36] J March, "What Constitutes a Stressor? The 'Criterion A' Issue" and J Davidson and J Fairbank, "The Epidemiology of Posttraumatic Stress Disorder" in J Davidson and E Foa (eds), *Posttraumatic Stress Disorder: DSM-IV and Beyond* (1993) p 37 at pp 39-40 and p 147 at pp 159-161 respectively; and B Green, "Defining Trauma: Terminology and Generic Stressor Dimensions" (1990) 20 Journal of Applied and Social Psychology 1632, 1634-1639. However, Breslau and Davis point to studies which show that PTSD symptoms may follow ordinary life stressors and cases in which all the other PTSD criteria are met but the stressor is not the "right" (that is, extreme) kind to warrant a diagnosis of PTSD at present: N Breslau and G Davis, "Posttraumatic Stress Disorder: The Stressor Criterion" (1987) 175 Journal of Nervous and Mental Disease 255, 259. Breslau and Davis call into question the existence of a qualitatively separate category for PTSD stressors and for other stressful, more common life events. They maintain that there is no direct support for two distinct classes in terms of their probability of bringing forth distress or disaster: *ibid*, 262. See also M Horowitz, G Bonanno and A Holen, "Pathological Grief: Diagnosis and explanation" (1993) 55 Psychosomatic Medicine 260, 269-271.

[37] See J March, "What Constitutes a Stressor? The 'Criterion A' Issue" in J Davidson and E Foa (eds), *Posttraumatic Stress Disorder: DSM-IV and Beyond* (1993) p 37 at pp 37-38.

[38] J March, *ibid*, pp 46-47.

[39] See, for example, N Breslau and G Davis, "Posttraumatic Stress Disorder: The Stressor Criterion" (1987) 175 Journal of Nervous and Mental Disease 255, 262. C B Scrignar, *Posttraumatic Stress Disorder: Diagnosis, Treatment, and Legal Issues* (2nd ed 1988) p 13 speaks of "vulnerable" individuals. See also Scrignar, *op cit*, pp 84-85. The link between predisposition and the development of psychiatric disorder, in particular PTSD following trauma, has been studied by a large number of researchers. See, for example, H Resnick, D Kilpatrick, C Best and T Kramer, "Vulnerability Stress Factors in Development of Posttraumatic Stress Disorder" (1992) 180 Journal of Nervous and Mental Disease 424.

[40] See J Davidson and J Fairbank, "The Epidemiology of Posttraumatic Stress Disorder" in J Davidson and E Foa (eds), *Posttraumatic Stress Disorder: DSM-IV and Beyond* (1993) p 147 at pp 161-162 and J Davidson and E Foa, Epilogue, *ibid*, p 229 at pp 229-230 respectively; and H Resnick, D Kilpatrick, C Best and T Kramer, "Vulnerability-Stress Factors in Development of Posttraumatic Stress Disorder" (1992) 180 Journal of Nervous and Mental Disease 424; W True et al, "A Twin Study of Genetic and Environmental Contributions to Liability for Posttraumatic Stress Symptoms" (1993) 50 Archives of General Psychiatry 257; E Schwarz and J Kowalski, "Personality Characteristics and Posttraumatic Stress Symptoms after a School Shooting" (1992) 180 Journal of Nervous and Mental Disease 735; and E W McCranie, L Hyer, P Boudewyns and M Woods, "Negative Parenting Behavior, Combat Exposure, and PTSD Symptom Severity. Test of a Person-Event Interaction Model" (1992) 180 Journal of Nervous and Mental Disease 431.

worth noting that, according to some of the literature, a major risk factor for the development of PTSD, including among those who are secondary victims, is the witnessing of a particularly horrific scene.[41]

(3) Prevalence and statistical probability

3.10   Although there is some difference of opinion in the literature, there has been an increasing body of empirical research into the development of PTSD, and this provides useful information about the incidence of psychiatric disorder in people exposed to trauma. Estimates of the incidence of such disorder have also been made on the basis of clinical experience. It has been estimated that an extreme event in which people are involved, for example, an air crash or a rape, is likely to give rise to PTSD in a majority of the survivors or victims.[42] This is in line with the

[41]   Along with life threat and physical injury March identifies grotesquery as possibly a major risk factor for the development of PTSD: J March, "What Constitutes a Stressor? The 'Criterion A' Issue" in J Davidson and E Foa (eds), *Posttraumatic Stress Disorder: DSM-IV and Beyond* (1993) p 37 at p 50. Similarly, Raphael and Middleton identify the severity of the stress or trauma to which the victim is exposed, particularly in terms of gruesomeness, as an important factor in the development of post-traumatic responses: B Raphael and W Middleton, "After the horror" (1988) 296 BMJ 1142, 1143. A study of road accident victims found that the principal and very strong predictor of post-traumatic syndromes was the rating of "horrific" intrusive memories of the accident: R Mayou, B Bryant and R Duthie, "Psychiatric consequences of road traffic accidents" (1993) 307 BMJ 647. In a study of the psychological trauma caused to fire fighters involved in a bushfire disaster, McFarlane and Papay found that the group of subjects who were diagnosed as suffering only from PTSD had sustained property loss significantly greater than those who developed an associated disorder, often involving the death and injury of livestock which had had to be killed and buried in particularly distressing and grotesque circumstances: A McFarlane and P Papay, "Multiple Diagnoses in Posttraumatic Stress Disorder in the Victims of a Natural Disaster" (1992) 180 Journal of Nervous and Mental Disease 498, 502. See also A McFarlane "The Longitudinal Course of Posttraumatic Morbidity: The Range of Outcomes and Their Predictors" (1988) 176 Journal of Nervous and Mental Disease 30, 35. In a study of Falklands war veterans, O'Brien and Hughes found a strong link between degree of combat exposure and development of PTSD. Veterans who were diagnosed with PTSD were more likely to have actively assisted in the management of casualties or to have lost friends through wounding or death, or to have killed the enemy: L O'Brien and S Hughes, "Symptoms of Posttraumatic Stress Disorder in Falklands Veterans Five Years After the Conflict" (1991) 159 British Journal of Psychiatry 135, 138. With regard to crime, a significant association has similarly been found between crime stress level exposure and the development of PTSD: H Resnick, D Kilpatrick, C Best and T Kramer, "Vulnerability-Stress Factors in Development of Posttraumatic Stress Disorder" (1992) 180 Journal of Nervous and Mental Disease 424, 428.

[42]   Air crashes: B Green, "Disasters and Posttraumatic Stress Disorder" in J Davidson and E Foa (eds), *Posttraumatic Stress Disorder: DSM-IV and Beyond* (1993) p 75 at pp 90-91 (65% of survivors); G Mezey, "Assessing Emotional and Psychological Harm and PTSD" in "Shock, Pain and Trauma: Psychiatric Aspects of Civil Litigation" (MIND conference, February 1993) p 4 (90% of survivors). Rape victims: D Kilpatrick and H Resnick, "Posttraumatic Stress Disorder Associated with Exposure to Criminal Victimisation in Clinical and Community Populations" in J Davidson and E Foa (eds), *Posttraumatic Stress Disorder: DSM-IV and Beyond* (1993) p 147 esp at pp 122-124 (57.1% in community based samples to 70-95% in agency referred samples). A recent survey of the major studies into the prevalence of disorders after traumatic events concludes that about 20% of the people that go through severely distressing events develop severe disorders: this survey is reviewed in D Brom, R Kleber and E Witztum, "The Prevalence of Posttraumatic Psychopathology in the General and the Clinical Population" (1991) 28 Israel Journal of Psychiatry and Related Sciences 53. The finding, however, also implied that 70-80% of

prevailing view that certain extreme types of traumatic event are likely to induce PTSD in most people (at least initially), regardless of predisposition.[43]

3.11   Research also suggests that between 30% and 60% of the people involved in natural disasters may develop PTSD, and even more may do so after man made disasters.[44] This may be the case even with firefighters, ambulance personnel and others who are trained to deal with emergencies and disasters: for example, a study of Australian firefighters involved in serious bushfires found prevalence rates of 32%, 27% and 30% at 4, 11 and 29 months after the exposure.[45] In relation to smaller scale and generally less overwhelming traumas, it has been estimated that a mugging might give rise to PTSD in 30% of the victims,[46] and a study of people presenting themselves for treatment for road traffic accident injury at a hospital accident department found that PTSD occurred in 11% of these victims during the year following the accident.[47] This study found a greater incidence of other conditions

people who go through such events cope with them in a successful manner: *ibid*, 57. Similarly, Breslau and Davis maintain that reports show that although most people display signs of emotional disturbance immediately after a disaster, this subsides and the rate of long-term disturbance is actually low: N Breslau and G Davis, "Posttraumatic Stress Disorder: The Stressor Criterion" (1987) 175 Journal of Nervous and Mental Disease 255, 261.

[43]   See para 3.9 n 40 above.

[44]   See B Raphael and W Middleton, "After the horror" (1988) 296 BMJ 1142, 1143 (citing the results of studies reported by A McFarlane, paras 3.13-3.14 and n 252 below); J Titchener and F Kapp, "Family and Character Change at Buffalo Creek" (1976) 133 American Journal of Psychiatry 295; cf S Madakasira and K O'Brien, "Acute Posttraumatic Stress Disorder in Victims of a Natural Disaster" (1987) 175 Journal of Nervous and Mental Disease 286, 289.

[45]   A McFarlane, "The Aetiology of Post-Traumatic Morbidity: Predisposing, Precipitating and Perpetuating Factors" (1989) 154 British Journal of Psychiatry 221, 223; A McFarlane, "Posttraumatic Morbidity of a Disaster: A Study of Cases Presenting for Psychiatric Treatment" (1986) 174 Journal of Nervous and Mental Disease 4; A McFarlane, "Life Events and Psychiatric Disorder: The Role of a Natural Disaster" (1987) 151 British Journal of Psychiatry 362; A McFarlane, "The Longitudinal Course of Posttraumatic Morbidity: The Range of Outcomes and their Predictors" (1988) 176 Journal of Nervous and Mental Disease 30; A McFarlane and P Papay, "Multiple Diagnoses in Posttraumatic Stress Disorder in the Victims of a Natural Disaster" (1992) 180 Journal of Nervous and Mental Disease 498. Cf D Alexander and A Wells, "Reactions of Police Officers to Body-Handling After a Major Disaster" (1991) 159 British Journal of Psychiatry 547.

[46]   G Mezey, "Assessing Emotional and Psychological Harm and PTSD" in "Shock, Pain and Trauma: Psychiatric Aspects of Civil Litigation" (MIND conference, February 1993) p 4.

[47]   R Mayou, B Bryant and R Duthie, "Psychiatric consequences of road traffic accidents" (1993) 307 BMJ 647, 649. See also L Sparr and J Boehnlein, "Posttraumatic Stress Disorder in Tort Actions: Forensic Minefield" (1990) 18 Bull Am Acad Psychiatry Law 283, 293, who cite one study of 100 litigation cases following car accidents in which fewer than 10 patients seemed to meet the criteria for PTSD. In a review of the literature on the psychological consequences of motor vehicle accidents, W Koch concluded that the base rate for PTSD subsequent to motor vehicle accidents associated with serious physical injury is greater than 10%, and that there may be other less severe psychological problems occurring in up to 33% of victims: "Post Traumatic Stress Disorder Subsequent to Motor Vehicle Accidents" (1994) 52 The Advocate 51, 52.

attributable to the accident, including phobic anxiety disorders, which were severe enough to be classified as psychiatric disorders by the standard diagnostic criteria.[48] It concluded that psychiatric symptoms and disorder in the aftermath of both major and less severe road accident injury are frequently to be found, and that post-traumatic stress symptoms were also common.[49] Significantly, in these road traffic accident cases, anxiety and depression were closely associated with evidence of pre-accident psychological or social problems. Post-traumatic stress symptoms, on the other hand, were unrelated to evidence of neurotic predisposition or previous emotional problems, but were strongly associated with initial horrific memories of the accident.[50]

3.12 The different reactions of children and adults to traumatic events has caused problems in diagnosing the reactions of children to traumatic events;[51] the difficulty in part arising from the fact that the criteria for disorders such as PTSD were not developed on the basis of studies of young people.[52] A 1993 review of research studies on children nevertheless concluded that PTSD was common following exposure to warfare, criminal violence, burns and serious accidents, but was less consistently found as a consequence of sexual abuse.[53] Although this review also concluded that there was little evidence that natural disasters *routinely* produced

---

[48] Evidence suggests that anxiety and depressive states are in fact the most common psychological reactions to traumatic events: Beebe (1975), Levav and Abramson (1984), Eaton et al (1982) and Tennant et al (1986) - cited in M Weller, "Compensation for psychiatric disability" in R Bluglass and P Bowden (eds), *Principles and Practice of Forensic Psychiatry* (1990) p 1101 at p 1105. See also B Green, J Lindy, M Grace and A Leonard, "Chronic Posttraumatic Stress Disorder and Diagnostic Comorbidity in a Disaster Sample" (1992) 180 Journal of Nervous and Mental Disease 760; L Goldberg and M Gara, "A Typology of Psychiatric Reactions to Motor Vehicle Accidents" (1990) 23 Psychopathology 15. McFarlane's study of bush fire-fighters in Australia showed that many who subsequently suffered from symptoms of PTSD suffered from chronic pain syndromes, depression and specific phobias. See also A McFarlane, "Posttraumatic Morbidity of a Disaster: A Study of Cases Presenting for Psychiatric Treatment" (1986) 174 Journal of Nervous and Mental Disease 4.

[49] R Mayou, B Bryant and R Duthie, "Psychiatric Consequences of Road Traffic Accidents" (1993) 307 BMJ 647. See also M Trimble, *Post-Traumatic Neurosis: From Railway Spine to the Whiplash* (1981) p 113 and studies cited therein.

[50] In a study of the prevalence of psychiatric illness among a population of firefighters exposed to a natural disaster, it was found that the subjects who were only suffering from PTSD appeared to have experienced the highest degree of exposure to the disaster. Of those who were diagnosed with other concurrent disorders such as depression and anxiety disorders, in addition to PTSD, it was found that adversity experienced both before and after the disaster influenced the onset of these disorders: A McFarlane and P Papay, "Multiple Diagnoses in Posttraumatic Stress Disorder in the Victims of a Natural Disaster" (1992) 180 Journal of Nervous and Mental Disease 498.

[51] N Garmezy and M Rutter, "Acute Reactions to Stress" in M Rutter and L Hersov (eds), *Child and Adolescent Psychiatry: Modern Approaches* (2nd ed 1985) p 152.

[52] W Yule, "Posttraumatic Stress Disorders" in M Rutter, E Taylor and L Hersov (eds) *Child and Adolescent Psychiatry: Modern Approaches* (3rd ed 1994) p 392 at p 394.

[53] R McNally, "Stressors that produce PTSD in Children" in J Davidson and E Foa (eds), *Posttraumatic Stress Disorder: DSM-IV and Beyond* (1993) ch 4.

PTSD in children, it accepted that specific events that can occur during a natural disaster (such as witnessing the death of a family member) may trigger off PTSD. On the other hand two other studies that were not apparently included in this review have estimated that after major disasters (such as those involving the "Herald of Free Enterprise" ferry and the school ship "Jupiter"), as many as 30-50% of the children involved will show significant symptomatology.[54] It has been said that of the survivors of the school ship "Jupiter" approximately 50% suffered from PTSD.[55] Studies of children who had been exposed to the experience of witnessing a parent being murdered[56] or sexually assaulted[57] found that they all suffered from PTSD. One study of children in a school playground who had been exposed to attack from a sniper found that 77% developed moderate or severe PTSD,[58] although another study found that only 27% were suffering from PTSD 6 to 14 months after a school shooting.[59]

3.13   Research studies also provide interesting, but perhaps unsurprising, material on the relevance to PTSD of physical injury and proximity.[60] Thus, for example, while one study found that 20% of wounded Vietnam veterans developed full PTSD, only 4% of non-wounded veterans developed the disorder.[61] Another study, of women who had been the victims of sexual assaults, found PTSD in 14.2% of those with physical injuries but in only 0.64% of those who had not been physically injured.[62] A study of children affected by the attack of a sniper in their school playground found that while 48.6% of children in the playground experienced severe PTSD,

---

[54]   The literature is reviewed in: W Yule, "Children in Shipping Disasters" (1991) 84 Journal of the Royal Society of Medicine 12, 13.

[55]   W Yule, "Post-Traumatic Stress Disorder in Child Survivors of Shipping Disasters: The Sinking of the 'Jupiter'" (1992) 57 Journal of Psychotherapy and Psychosomatics 200, 204 (2nd European Conference on Traumatic Stress).

[56]   C P Malmquist, "Children Who Witness Parental Murder: Posttraumatic Aspects" (1986) 25 Journal of the American Academy of Child and Adolescent Psychiatry 320.

[57]   R Pynoos and K Nader, "Children who Witness the Sexual Assaults of Their Mothers" (1988) 27 Journal of the American Academy of Child and Adolescent Psychiatry 567.

[58]   R Pynoos et al, "Life Threat and Posttraumatic Stress in School-age Children" (1987) 44 Archives of General Psychiatry 1057, 1059.

[59]   E Schwarz and J Kowalski, "Malignant Memories: PTSD in Children and Adults after a School Shooting" (1991) 30 Journal of the American Academy of Child and Adolescent Psychiatry 936 (27% of children and 19% of adults met the criteria for PTSD 6 to 14 months after the shooting. No distinction was made regarding the location of the children at the time of the shooting).

[60]   J Davidson and J Fairbank review a number of studies in "The Epidemiology of Posttraumatic Stress Disorder" in J Davidson and E Foa (eds), *Posttraumatic Stress Disorder: DSM-IV and Beyond* (1993) p 147 at pp 159-161.

[61]   J Helzer, L Robins and L McEvoy, "Post-Traumatic Stress Disorder in the General Population" (1987) 317 New England Journal of Medicine 1630, 1632.

[62]   I Winfield, L George, M Swartz and D Blazer, "Sexual Assault and Psychiatric Disorders among a Community Sample of Women" (1990) 147 American Journal of Psychiatry 335.

only 16.7% of those at school suffered such a degree of PTSD and this level fell to 7% for those who were not at school at the time. Similarly, 55.8% of the children not at school did not suffer from PTSD at all but of those in the playground only 5.7% did not experience any form of PTSD.[63]

3.14   A number of community-based surveys have found that the prevalence of a history of PTSD in the general population ranges from between 1% and 2.6%. Its incidence rises to between 3.3% and 6.3% in various risk groups which have been exposed to unusual and distressing trauma (for example, combat veterans).[64]

3.15   It is clear that these studies, taken as a whole, are open to more than one interpretation and that, indeed, different surveys have produced different findings. It is also important to note that the studies were compiled primarily for treatment and research purposes and that they do not give any indication of the proportion of those who develop PTSD or related psychiatric injury following trauma who then seek compensation for their injury, nor the proportion of those whose claims are likely to succeed. Furthermore, although a serious threat of harm to one's spouse, children, close relatives or friends (or the *learning* of such a threat) can be the basis of a diagnosis of PTSD,[65] most of the studies are concerned with situations in which the psychiatric illness was suffered by people who were themselves exposed to risk.[66] Nevertheless, we would suggest that the literature and surveys can be fairly interpreted as lending support to three views that have been, or ought to be, significant in shaping the law, namely that:

> (1)   Psychiatry does recognise a distinction between mere mental distress and psychiatric illness although this may be a matter of degree rather than kind.

> (2)   Those who are themselves injured or at risk of injury or, probably, are physically proximate to a traumatic event are more likely to suffer shock-induced psychiatric illness than those who are not; on the other hand, it is recognised that shock-induced psychiatric illness may be

---

[63]   R Pynoos et al, "Life Threat and Posttraumatic Stress in School-age Children" (1987) 44 Archives of General Psychiatry 1057, 1059.

[64]   J Davidson and J Fairbank, "The Epidemiology of Posttraumatic Stress Disorder" in J Davidson and E Foa (eds), *Posttraumatic Stress Disorder: DSM-IV and Beyond* (1993) p 147 esp at p 150. See also J Helzer, L Robins and L McEvoy, "Post-Traumatic Stress Disorder in the General Population" (1987) 317 New England Journal of Medicine 1630.

[65]   Paras 3.5, 3.7 and 3.8 above.

[66]   Ie in general they do not deal with the most legally controversial area of "secondary victims": but see the studies of children following a sniper's attack or witnessing a parent being murdered, in paras 3.12 and 3.13 above and of bush firefighters in para 3.11 above. Also see T Newburn, "The Long-Term Needs of Victims: A Review of the Literature", Research and Planning Unit Paper 80, Home Office, pp 10-13 (dealing with the indirect victims of crime).

suffered by a family member or close friend who learns about an injury or unexpected death to another.

(3) There is a serious risk that the floodgates of litigation would be opened if the sole test for liability in negligence was whether it was reasonably foreseeable that psychiatric illness would be caused to the plaintiff.

3.16 **We invite consultees to bear this brief summary of recent medical research in mind when they are considering the options for reform in Part V of this paper and we would also welcome any general comments on it. More specifically, we invite the views of those with expertise in the field: (a) as to whether they consider that our summary of the relevant medical background and research, and our conclusions, are fair and accurate and, if not, why not; (b) as to what they believe to be the incidence of psychiatric illnesses caused by injury to, or fear for the safety of, others and as to whether a survey could sensibly be carried out on that specific issue; and (c) as to any other medical considerations they believe we should be taking into account.**

PART IV
POLICY ARGUMENTS FOR LIMITING RECOVERY

4.1 A number of policy-based arguments may be advanced to justify a cautious approach to recovery for psychiatric illness where this is not parasitic on some other personal injury suffered by the plaintiff. These may be based on a fear of the "floodgates" opening, a concern about fraudulent and exaggerated claims, problems about conflicting medical opinions, a feeling that psychiatric illness is less serious than bodily injury, and the fact that the plaintiff is commonly only a secondary victim. We will consider each of these arguments in turn.

(Page v Smith)

(1) Fear of the "floodgates" opening[1]

4.2 The cautious approach of the courts in cases involving pure economic loss is said to have had its origins in a fear of the impossibility of containing liability within any acceptable bounds. This is often called the "floodgates" argument.[2] The opportunities for the infliction of pecuniary loss from the negligent performance of everyday tasks are very wide, since the effects of such negligence "are illimitable and the effects are far-reaching."[3] The floodgates argument has also traditionally been used to support a restrictive approach towards recovery for psychiatric illness because "shock" is in its nature capable of affecting a similarly wide range of persons.[4] The floodgates argument is primarily based on the fear of a proliferation of claims from a single event, although it is also sometimes used to refer to the fear of many claims from a mass of separate events. Such a proliferation would clog up the court system and divert too many of society's resources into compensating the victims of psychiatric illness at the expense of the many who presently receive little or no compensation, even for physical injuries suffered as a result of negligent conduct.[5] If the burden of cost is too great it cannot and will not be met, the law

---

[1] Sir Richard Couch, delivering the judgment of the Privy Council in *Victorian Railways Comrs v Coultas* (1888) 13 App Cas 222, 225-226, said that "in every case where an accident caused by negligence had given a person a serious nervous shock there might be a claim for damages on account of mental injury. The difficulty which now often exists in a case of alleged physical injuries of determining whether they were caused by the negligent act would be greatly increased, and a wide field opened for imaginary claims". The influence of the "floodgates" argument upon the development of liability for psychiatric illness is discussed by Hidden J at first instance in *Alcock v Chief Constable of South Yorkshire Police* [1992] 1 AC 310, 331ff; and all their Lordships in *Alcock* refer to it as a major reason for their restrictive approach. See also J G Fleming, "Remoteness and Duty: the Control Devices in Liability for Negligence" (1953) 31 Can BR 471, 492-493; G L Fricke, "Nervous Shock - the Opening of the Floodgates" (1981) 7 Univ of Tasmania LR 113; N J Mullany and P R Handford, *op cit*, pp 311-314.

[2] *Murphy v Brentwood District Council* [1991] 1 AC 398, 485, *per* Lord Oliver.

[3] *Caparo Industries Plc v Dickman* [1990] 2 AC 605, 632, *per* Lord Oliver.

[4] See *McLoughlin v O'Brian* [1983] 1 AC 410, 422, *per* Lord Wilberforce; 424, *per* Lord Edmund-Davies.

[5] *Atiyah's Accidents, Compensation and the Law* (5th ed 1993) p 73.

will fall into disrepute, and it will be a disservice to victims who might reasonably have expected compensation.[6] The floodgates objection also rests on the notion that to allow a mass of claims from a single event would be unfair to the defendant and would impose a burden disproportionate to the negligent conduct complained of. Fairness to the defendant is in turn linked to concerns about the impact of awards on insurance. The cost of liability is spread by insurance and any large additional burden on insurers will be ultimately borne by those who are insured, in particular road users and employers, but also consumers and, in the case of defendants which are public authorities, taxpayers.[7]

4.3   Although the force of the floodgates objection has been disputed by some judges both in this area[8] and in relation to negligently caused pure economic loss,[9] the courts continue to be influenced by it. In *Alcock* the speeches acknowledge the argument as the reason for the general approach the courts have adopted to claims for "nervous shock".[10]

4.4   The particular fact situation in *Alcock*, a large scale disaster broadcast on national television, made it clear to the House of Lords that the application of the ordinary "reasonable foreseeability" test for the existence of a duty of care in personal injury cases could lead to a high number of claims. Television viewers in particular were seen as representing a dangerously large category of potential claimants, in view of the increasing ability of the media to show live coverage of disasters or accidents. Similarly, people who sustain psychiatric illness as a result of being told about an incident constitute a potentially large category of possible claimants.

4.5   Renewed fear of the floodgates opening has been fuelled in part by the psychiatric profession's refinement of its perception of post-traumatic stress reactions or disorders, and by a greater willingness by doctors to support such claims.[11] PTSD in particular has captured the imagination of both psychiatrists and lawyers, and it

---

[6]   *McLoughlin v O'Brian* [1983] 1 AC 410, 425, *per* Lord Edmund-Davies, citing Griffiths LJ in the Court of Appeal [1981] QB 599, 623.

[7]   See eg *Wise v Kaye* [1962] 1 QB 638, 670, *per* Diplock LJ; *Fletcher v Autocar and Transporters Ltd* [1968] 2 QB 322, 335-336, *per* Lord Denning MR; *Hansard* (HC) 3 March 1989, vol 148, cols 515, 527-528 (Mr Stanley Orme MP, Mr Lawrence Cunliffe MP and Mr James Arbuthnot MP). For discussion of these considerations in the context of economic loss, see Lord Oliver, "Developments in Professional Liability" (Chartered Insurance Institute, 1988); P Cane, *Tort Law and Economic Interests* (1991) pp 441-446. See also *Hansard* (HL) 18 March 1987, vol 485, cols 1463-7 (Lord Hacking).

[8]   See, eg, *McLoughlin v O'Brian* [1983] 1 AC 410, 442, *per* Lord Bridge.

[9]   *Junior Books Ltd v Veitchi Co Ltd* [1983] 1 AC 520.

[10]   [1992] 1 AC 310, 419, *per* Lord Jauncey; 410, 417, *per* Lord Oliver; 401-402, *per* Lord Ackner; 396-397, *per* Lord Keith.

[11]   See J Swanton, "Issues in Tort Liability for Nervous Shock" (1992) 66 ALJ 495, 497; C Pugh and M Trimble, "Psychiatric Injury after Hillsborough" (1993) 163 British Journal of Psychiatry 425, 426.

is now considered as a matter of course when assessing potential claims for compensation in a wide variety of situations apart from disasters.[12] New diagnostic categories of psychiatric illness have been proposed, and the concept of psychiatric illness has widened significantly in recent years.[13] Moreover there is no longer any shame or disgrace attached to seeking psychiatric treatment, or admitting that one is suffering from mental illness.[14]

4.6   It has been argued, however, that fears of the floodgates opening may be misplaced.[15] It is said, for example, that the requirement of proof that the plaintiff is suffering from a recognised psychiatric illness is, in itself, a considerable hurdle to surmount.[16] We have explained that two diagnostic classificatory systems ("DSM" and "ICD") have been developed which broadly represent consensus views of the psychiatric profession as to the conditions from which patients are suffering.[17] All the legitimate diagnoses of psychiatric conditions today must meet the diagnostic criteria which are contained in the current versions of one or other of these two

---

[12]   M Napier, "The medical and legal response to post-traumatic stress disorder" in A Grubb (ed), *Choices and Decisions in Health Care* (1993) p 205, at p 206; M Weller, "Post traumatic stress disorder" (1993) 143 NLJ 878. See para 3.5 above.

[13]   The diagnosis "Acute Stress Disorder" is new in DSM-IV and was added to describe acute reactions to extreme stress (ie, occurring within 4 weeks of the stressor and lasting from 2 days to 4 weeks): para 308.3, 429-432 and Appendix D, p 783. It has also been suggested that there is evidence to support the existence of a more complex stress reaction than PTSD occurring characteristically in victims of prolonged, repeated interpersonal violence or victimisation: J Herman, "Sequelae of Prolonged and Repeated Trauma: Evidence for a Complex Posttraumatic Syndrome (DESNOS)" in J Davidson and E Foa (eds), *Posttraumatic Stress Disorder: DSM-IV and Beyond* (1993) ch 12. However, Pugh and Trimble have suggested that the extension of stress-related syndromes to much broader categories is likely to create further confusion in the medico-legal setting: C Pugh and M Trimble, "Psychiatric Injury after Hillsborough" (1993) 163 British Journal of Psychiatry 425, 429. The need has also been stressed for a new diagnosis of symptoms precipitated by a loss event such as bereavement (which is virtually a universal experience and thus will not suffice for a diagnosis of PTSD): M Horowitz, G Bonanno and A Holen, "Pathological Grief: Diagnosis and Explanation" (1993) 55 Psychosomatic Medicine 260.

[14]   J Swanton, "Issues in Tort Liability for Nervous Shock" (1992) 66 ALJ 495, 497.

[15]   See N J Mullany and P R Handford, *op cit*, pp 312-314. See also B S Markesinis and S F Deakin, *Tort Law* (3rd ed 1994) pp 122-123; K J Nasir, "Nervous Shock and *Alcock*: The Judicial Buck Stops Here" (1992) 55 MLR 705, 713; H Teff, "The Hillsborough Football Disaster and Claims for 'Nervous Shock'" (1992) 32 Med Sci Law 251, 254; H Teff, "Liability for Negligently Inflicted Nervous Shock" (1983) 99 LQR 100, 105-106; J Steele, "Scepticism and the Law of Negligence" [1993] CLJ 437, 449-450; A Gore, correspondence (1994) 57 MLR 174.

[16]   N J Mullany and P R Handford, *op cit*, p 312; See also B Raphael and W Middleton, "After the horror" (1988) 296 BMJ 1142, 1143; L Sparr and J Boehnlein, "Posttraumatic Stress Disorder in Tort Actions: Forensic Minefield" (1990) 18 Bull Am Acad Psychiatry Law 283, 292.

[17]   See Part III above.

systems: DSM-IV or ICD-10.[18] Any discrepancy between the diagnosis and either of the diagnostic systems can be probed in court in cross-examination, as can any failure to consider or rule out alternative causes or factors in the plaintiff's life that could account for the complaint.[19] Other factors which have been identified as militating against a flood of claims include the strain of adversarial proceedings leading to a court appearance. In addition, a claimant might well receive medical advice not to proceed with a claim given that the time-scale of litigation does not correspond with that of the healing process where emotional stress is involved. And it may be that the "secondary" nature of most claims means that this is an area where claims-consciousness and social expectations are unusually weak at present.[20]

(2) Fraudulent and exaggerated claims

4.7   Judicial caution in this area may be attributable in part to the fear of a proliferation of groundless or exaggerated claims.[21] In particular, the danger of exaggerated claims has been described as the only real problem that "nervous shock" poses for the courts.[22] More specifically, the fear may be first, that claimants can relatively easily fake the "symptoms" of a psychiatric illness; and secondly, that even if the courts might not be taken in by fraudulent and exaggerated claims, it may not be easy to challenge such claims without coming to court so that out-of-court settlements will be hampered. A further linked point is that there may be a feeling that plaintiffs can easily exploit the legitimate differences of opinion that exist within the psychiatric profession.[23]

[18]   For a brief but helpful description of the scales used for "scoring" PTSD - and literature on this issue - see J Shepherd, P Richmond and D Miers, "Assessing General Damages: A Medical Model" (1994) 144 NLJ 162, 163-164. See also M Horowitz, N Wilner and W Alvarez, "Impact of Event Scale: A Measure of Subjective Stress" (1979) 41 Psychosomatic Medicine 209. Note that worries have been expressed about the dangers of a "checklist" approach to diagnosis: see L Sparr and J Boehnlein, "Posttraumatic Stress Disorder in Tort Actions: Forensic Minefield" (1990) 18 Bull Am Acad Psychiatry Law 283, 290-292 and articles cited therein; W Yule, "Posttraumatic Stress Disorders" in M Rutter, E Taylor and L Herzov (eds), *Child and Adolescent Psychiatry: Modern Approaches* (3rd ed 1994) p 392 at p 403.

[19]   See S B Bisbing, "Challenging Psychological Damages Claims in Civil Litigation" (1992) 59 Def Couns J 358.

[20]   H Teff, "Liability for Negligently Inflicted Nervous Shock" (1983) 99 LQR 100, 111-112.

[21]   *McLoughlin v O'Brian* [1983] 1 AC 410, 421, *per* Lord Wilberforce; 442, *per* Lord Bridge. In *Victorian Railways Commissioners v Coultas* this was given as a reason for an absolute refusal to recognise nervous shock claims: (1888) 13 App Cas 222, 226, *per* Sir Richard Couch.

[22]   J S Williams, "Torts - Nervous Shock - Relation to Nominate Torts" (1968) 46 Can BR 515.

[23]   See para 4.10 below.

4.8   This fear, however, has for the most part been derided by the courts.[24]   The requirement that the plaintiff must establish a recognised psychiatric illness will in itself provide a deterrent to trivial claims and some deterrent to fraudulent claims. Moreover, although many psychiatric illnesses (for example, PTSD) cannot be substantiated by "physical" tests (such as blood tests), a number of psychological tests now exist which can help to ascertain whether the plaintiff has faked or exaggerated psychological symptoms and whether he or she is a credible informant.[25] These tests also distinguish long-standing character problems and dysfunctions from illness or injury of sudden onset. The tests are objective and are often given and scored by computer. They are complemented by clinical evaluation, by an examination of the person's pre- and post-accident functioning, and by corroborative interviews with family members.[26]

4.9   One commentator has argued that psychiatrists and psychologists are susceptible to deception. This was demonstrated in a study he undertook in which psychiatrists were tricked into incorrect diagnoses.[27] However, criticism has been levied against the method used in the study, and against its analysis and conclusions.[28] Although we are aware that allegations of feigned psychosis or actual fabrication are still made in contested litigation, the medical literature suggests that it is not common.[29]

---

[24]   See, for example, *Bourhill v Young* 1941 SC 395, 438. In *McLoughlin v O'Brian* [1983] 1 AC 410, 421 Lord Wilberforce thought that a fear of fraudulent claims should not inhibit the development of the law with respect to claims for psychiatric injury. He considered that these could be contained by the courts, which could also cope with any evidentiary difficulties. See also M Davie, "Negligently Inflicted Psychiatric Illness: The Hillsborough Case in the House of Lords" (1992) 43 NILQ 237, 248-249.

[25]   See C B Scrignar, *Posttraumatic Stress Disorder: Diagnosis, Treatment, and Legal Issues* (2nd ed 1988) pp 142-145. See also para 4.6 n 18 above. Criteria have been formulated by the psychiatric profession itself to determine whether a patient is malingering: DSM-IV, para V65.2, p 683. See M Weller, "Compensation for psychiatric disability" in R Bluglass and P Bowden (eds), *Principles and Practice of Forensic Psychiatry* (1990) p 1101 at p 1104.

[26]   See Comment, "Negligently Inflicted Mental Distress: The Case for an Independent Tort" [1971] 59 Georgetown LJ 1237, 1253, 1260 and 1261-1262. According to N J Mullany and P R Handford, *op cit*, p 310: "In the light of current psychological and psychiatric investigative techniques, the risk of fraud is miniscule. One suspects it is easier to fake or magnify a bad back than a psychiatrically imbalanced mind".

[27]   D Rosenhan, "On Being Sane in Insane Places" (1973) 179 Science 250.

[28]   See R Spitzer, "More on Pseudoscience in Science and the Case for Psychiatric Diagnosis" (1976) 33 Archives of General Psychiatry 459 and M Weller, "Compensation for psychiatric disability" in R Bluglass and P Bowden (eds), *Principles and Practice of Forensic Psychiatry* (1990) p 1101 at p 1103. See also S T Perconte, "Failure to Detect Fabricated Posttraumatic Stress Disorder with the use of the MMPI in a Clinical Population" (1990) 147 American Journal of Psychiatry 1057; L Sparr and L Pankratz, "Factitious Posttraumatic Stress Disorder" (1983) 140 American Journal of Psychiatry 1016; L Pankratz, "Continued Appearance of Factitious Posttraumatic Stress Disorder" (1990) 147 American Journal of Psychiatry 811.

[29]   See G Hay, "Feigned Psychosis: a Review of the Simulation of Mental Illness" (1983) 43 British Journal of Psychiatry 8, 10; P Lees-Haley, "Efficacy of MPI-2 Validity Scales and MCMI-II Modifier Scales for Detecting Spurious PTSD Claims" (1992) 48 Journal of Clinical Psychology 681. A recent study of 188 road traffic accident victims found that

(3) Conflicting medical opinions

4.10   As we have seen in Part III of this paper, there has been extensive research relating
to the phenomenon of traumatic stress reactions, and PTSD in particular, and a
consensus of opinion among experts dealing in this sphere is now evident from the
psychiatric and psychological literature.[30] However, differences may legitimately arise
between different medical experts[31] not merely as to the precise mental disorder
from which the plaintiff is suffering, but also as to its severity, its cause and the
future prognosis. Members of the psychiatric profession have themselves
acknowledged that the scientific basis of their knowledge and practice is neither
fixed nor universally agreed on.[32] Disagreement among mental health professionals
concerning the presence or absence of a mental disorder following trauma can
represent legitimate differences based on an honest assessment of the patient.[33]
There may be some judicial hostility to psychiatric expert evidence, attributable in
part to an awareness of the fluidity of psychiatric thinking compared with that
generally applied by the medical profession,[34] and also to a perception of psychiatry
as being a relatively new discipline. Moreover, concerns have been expressed about
bias in psychiatric expert evidence, in particular the willingness of some mental
health professionals to compromise themselves for fees as expert witnesses and agree
to a legally predetermined position.[35] It would seem, however, that while these
problems may assume greater significance in cases of psychiatric illness, there is

exaggeration or malingering was uncommon: R Mayou, B Bryant and R Duthie,
"Psychiatric consequences of road traffic accidents" (1993) 307 BMJ 647.

[30]   See paras 3.5-3.9 above. See also B S Markesinis and S F Deakin, *Tort Law* (3rd ed 1994)
p 121.

[31]   N Kreitman, "The reliability of psychiatric diagnosis" (1961) 107 Journal of Mental
Science 876 and N Kreitman et al, "The reliability of psychiatric diagnosis: an analysis"
(1961) 107 Journal of Mental Science 887; *Phipson on Evidence* (14th ed 1990), para 32-
40, p 831; B Hoffman and H Spiegel, "Legal Principles in the Psychiatric Assessment of
Personal Injury Litigants" (1989) 146 American Journal of Psychiatry 304, 308-309; C
Scrignar, *Post-Traumatic Stress Disorder: Diagnosis, Treatment and Legal Issues* (2nd ed 1988)
pp 220-221.

[32]   B Hoffman and H Spiegel, "Legal Principles in the Psychiatric Assessment of Personal
Injury Litigants" (1989) 146 American Journal of Psychiatry 304, 308-309.

[33]   C Scrignar, *Post-Traumatic Stress Disorder: Diagnosis, Treatment and Legal Issues* (2nd ed
1988) p 145.

[34]   See *McLoughlin v O'Brian* [1983] 1 AC 410, 432-433, *per* Lord Bridge.

[35]   See Sir George Jessel MR in *Lord Abinger v Ashton* (1873) LR 17 Eq 358, 373-374; *Joseph
Crosfield & Sons v Techno-Chemical Laboratories Ltd* (1913) 29 TLR 378, 379, *per* Neville J.
See also C Jones, *Expert Witnesses: Science, Medicine and the Practice of Law* (1994) pp 97-
102 and 126. This fear was adverted to by Lord Wilberforce in *McLoughlin v O'Brian*
[1983] 1 AC 410, 421, in his identification of the policy arguments against an extension of
the law beyond its then limits, when he referred to the possible "establishment of an
industry of lawyers and psychiatrists who will formulate a claim for nervous shock
damages...for all, or many, road accidents and industrial accidents". See also *Phipson on
Evidence* (14th ed 1990), para 32.40; C Scrignar, *Post-Traumatic Stress Disorder: Diagnosis,
Treatment and Legal Issues* (2nd ed 1988) pp 220-221; S Carne, "Expert Evidence" SJ
Supplement, 11 December 1992, 24; J Hall and G Smith, "Solicitors and Expert
Witnesses" SJ Supplement, 11 December 1992, 12.

ultimately no reason why the courts should be any less capable of weighing competing expert evidence in this sphere than in many other spheres. There is also evidence which shows that psychiatrists are as consistent in their diagnoses as other physicians.[36]

(4) Psychiatric illness is less serious than bodily injury

4.11 Mullany and Handford suggest that the most telling reason for the courts' restrictive approach to claims for psychiatric illness is that injury to the mind is thought less worthy of community and legal support than physical injury to the body.[37] They argue cogently, however, that the fact that such injury is not visible to the naked eye does not mean that it is not real, and that on one view the mental repercussions of trauma are more serious, and more deserving of the law's attention, than those of a physical nature: "as a general observation, an injured mind is far more difficult to nurse back to health than an injured body and is arguably more debilitating and disruptive of a greater number of aspects of human existence."[38] The seriousness of psychiatric illness has also been impressed upon us, on preliminary consultation, by medical and legal experts working in the field.[39]

(5) The plaintiff is commonly a secondary victim

4.12 In the standard case where the shock arose from an injury to, or fear for the safety of, another the plaintiff can be viewed as a secondary victim of the tortious conduct. One argument in favour of the restrictive approach which is applied to shock-induced psychiatric illness stems from a certain ambivalence about compensating such secondary victims.[40] In the words of Lord Oliver in *Alcock*, "[E]xcept in those cases which were based upon some ancient and now outmoded concepts of the quasi-proprietorial rights of husbands over their wives, parents over their children or employers over their menial servants, the common law has, in general, declined to entertain claims for such consequential injuries from third parties, save possibly where loss has arisen from the necessary performance of a legal duty imposed on such party by the injury to the victim".[41]

---

[36] Shepherd, Brooke, Cooper and Linn (1968) Acta Psychiatrica et Neurologica Scandinavia (suppl 201) 44 and Fletcher (1952) 45 Proceedings of the Royal Society of Medicine 577 cited by M Weller, "Compensation for psychiatric disability" in R Bluglass and P Bowden (eds), *Principles and Practice of Forensic Psychiatry* (1990) p 1101 at p 1103.

[37] *Tort Liability for Psychiatric Damage* (1993) p 309, citing Birkett J in *Griffiths v R & H Green and Silley Weir Ltd* (1948) 81 Ll L Rep 378, 380: see para 1.9 above.

[38] *Ibid*, p 323.

[39] See para 1.9 above.

[40] See H Teff, "Liability for negligently inflicted nervous shock" (1983) 99 LQR 100, 104; N J Mullany and P R Handford, *op cit*, ch 4.

[41] [1992] 1 AC 310, 409.

4.13 But as Lord Oliver also pointed out,[42] the description of the plaintiff in psychiatric illness cases as a "secondary victim" does not obviate the need to establish that the defendant owes a direct duty to the plaintiff.[43] It may be, therefore, that at root this "secondary victim" objection again rests on the fear of opening the floodgates of litigation in its main sense of there being a mass of claims from a single event. Moreover it clearly has no application where, as in some cases, the plaintiff is the primary victim.[44]

---

[42] [1992] 1 AC 310, 411. See also Lord Wright in *Bourhill v Young* [1943] AC 92, 108.

[43] It also follows from this that the contributory negligence of the primary victim does not lead to a reduction of the damages payable to the secondary victim. See para 5.50 below.

[44] See propositions (3), (5), (6) and (7) in para 2.3 above.

PART V
OPTIONS FOR REFORM

5.1   We have divided our discussion of the options for reform into seven main questions:
(1) should there no longer be liability for negligently inflicted "pure" psychiatric
illness?; (2) should it be a requirement that the psychiatric illness sustained by the
plaintiff be by reason of actual or apprehended physical injury to the plaintiff?; (3)
what should be the law where the defendant has negligently injured or imperilled
someone other than the plaintiff, and the plaintiff, as a result, has foreseeably
suffered a psychiatric illness?; (4) what should be the law where the defendant has
negligently damaged or imperilled property belonging to the plaintiff or to a third
party, and the plaintiff, as a result, has foreseeably suffered a psychiatric illness?; (5)
should there be liability for the negligent communication of news to the plaintiff
foreseeably causing him or her to suffer a psychiatric illness?; (6) should there be
liability where an employer has negligently overburdened an employee with work
thereby foreseeably causing him or her to suffer a psychiatric illness?; (7) is
legislation required in relation to negligently inflicted psychiatric illness?

5.2   Of these, the main controversy, in our view, relates to the third question which we
shall examine by asking a further nine questions. It is perhaps worth emphasising
at the outset, however, that three broad strategies may be adopted in relation to that
third question: (a) that the present law should be left as it is; (b) that psychiatric
illness (or, at least, shock-induced psychiatric illness) should be treated like any
other personal injury so that no special controls should apply; or (c) that some, but
not all, of the special controls should be removed, most obviously by abandoning
the present insistence on closeness in time and space and perception through one's
own unaided senses where the plaintiff has a close tie of love and affection to the
primary victim. As shall become clear, we provisionally favour the third, "mid-
position", strategy.

(1) Should there no longer be liability for negligently inflicted "pure" psychiatric illness?

5.3   The award of damages for negligently inflicted psychiatric illness is now well
established, albeit restricted. We consider that damages for this kind of harm serve
a genuine social need and that their award is correct in principle. We believe that
it is neither desirable nor realistic to return to the position (before *Dulieu v White*)[1]
when it was considered that there could be no liability for negligently inflicted pure
psychiatric illness. Having said that, there is a view, most cogently expressed by Jane
Stapleton,[2] that liability for negligently inflicted "nervous shock" should be wiped
away altogether because the boundaries that must be drawn to control liability are

---

[1]   [1901] 2 KB 669. See para 2.12 above.

[2]   J Stapleton, "In Restraint of Tort" in P Birks (ed), *Frontiers of Liability* (1994) vol 2, pp
94-96.

artificial and bring the law into disrepute. While we accept that some of the present controls may be artificial and may tend to bring the law into disrepute, we do not accept that all the possible controls are so tainted. **Our provisional view is that there should continue to be liability for negligently inflicted psychiatric illness that does not arise from a physical injury to the plaintiff. We ask consultees to say whether they agree with this provisional view. If they do not agree, please would they give their reasons.**

(2) Should it be a requirement that the psychiatric illness sustained by the plaintiff be by reason of actual or apprehended physical injury to the plaintiff?

5.4   Until the decision in *Hambrook v Stokes Bros*[3] negligence liability for psychiatric illness, not arising from personal injury, only existed in those cases where the illness resulted from the plaintiff's reasonably sustained fear for his or her own safety.[4] One possible reform would be to restrict liability to such cases, and to exclude cases where the psychiatric illness is sustained as the result of actual or apprehended personal injury to a third party. The requirement that the plaintiff is within the "zone of danger" is contained in the 1965 American Restatement (Second) of Torts and it is still the law in a substantial minority of United States jurisdictions.[5] And in some other jurisdictions, for example, Scotland, the courts have been slow to allow claims where this condition is not met.[6]

5.5   The reintroduction of this limit into English law would meet several of the policy objections to recovery we have noted.[7] For example, it would entirely negate the "secondary victim" argument.[8] It would also meet the floodgates objection,[9] since the number of potential plaintiffs from any incident would be very much reduced

---

[3]   [1925] 1 KB 141.

[4]   See paras 2.12-2.13 above.

[5]   Alabama; Arizona; Arkansas; Colorado; Delaware; District of Columbia; Georgia; Idaho; Illinois; Maryland; Minnesota; New York; North Carolina; North Dakota; Oklahoma; Oregon; South Dakota; Tennessee; Utah; Vermont; Virginia; Washington; West Virginia; Wisconsin. See D B Marlowe, "Negligent Infliction of Mental Distress" (1988) 33 Villanova Law Rev 781, 794-801; J Hwang, "Emotional Distress Law in Disarray" (1987) Annual Survey of American Law 475, 475-476 n 4; E McCarthy, "Illinois law in distress: the 'zone of danger' and 'physical injury' rules in emotional distress litigation" (1985) 19 J Marshall L Rev 17, 25. Reviewers arguing in favour of the zone of danger rule include D Crump, "Evaluating Independent Torts Based Upon 'Intentional' or 'Negligent' Infliction of Emotional Distress: How Can We Keep the Baby from Dissolving in the Bath Water?" (1992) 34 Ariz L Rev 439, and R Pearson, "Liability to Bystanders for Negligently Inflicted Emotional Harm - A Comment on the Nature of Arbitrary Rules" (1982) 34 U Fla L Rev 477.

[6]   See Appendix, para 1 below.

[7]   See Part IV above.

[8]   See paras 4.12-4.13 above.

[9]   See paras 4.2-4.6 above.

and it would only include those to whom a duty arose in respect of physical injury. The risk of fraudulent or exaggerated claims[10] might also be reduced, in that the medical literature and surveys suggest that those who are injured or at risk of injury (or, probably, are physically present at a traumatic event) are more likely to suffer shock-induced psychiatric illness than those who are not.[11]

5.6 Despite these advantages, subject to the views of consultees, we do not favour the reintroduction of a requirement of actual or apprehended physical injury to the plaintiff. To do so would exclude many deserving cases and would lead to distinctions which would be difficult to justify and would appear arbitrary. For example, to treat plaintiffs who think only of their own safety differently from those who, like the mothers in *Hambrook v Stokes Bros*[12] or *McLoughlin v O'Brian*,[13] are devoted to their family, would not be satisfactory. There are also strong policy reasons for not discouraging rescuers. Unless a special exception was introduced, the adoption of this limit would deny rescuers who suffer shock-induced psychiatric illness a right to recover compensation for their illness. **We ask consultees to say whether they agree with our provisional view that it should not be a requirement of liability that the psychiatric illness be sustained by reason of actual or apprehended physical injury to the plaintiff. If they do not agree, please would they give their reasons.**

---

[10] See paras 4.7-4.9 above.

[11] Para 3.13 above. L Goldberg and M Gara, "A Typology of Psychiatric Reactions to Motor Vehicle Accidents" (1990) 23 Psychopathology 15; B Green, "Defining Trauma: Terminology and Generic Stressor Dimensions" (1990) 20 Journal of Applied Social Psychology 1632, 1635; D Kilpatrick et al, "Criminal Victimization: lifetime prevalence, reporting to police, and psychological impact" (1987) 33 Crime and Delinquency 479; P Milici, "Postemotive Schizophrenia" (1939) 13 Psychiat Quart 278. See also, however, A Feinstein and R Dolan, "Post-traumatic stress disorder after physical trauma" (1991) 21 Psychological Medicine 85, 90 (the facts, in Feinstein and Dolan's study, that the traumatic event was life-threatening, and that the patient subjectively rated the severity of the trauma as being extremely high, did not appear to exert any lasting influence on the development of psychopathology).

[12] [1925] 1 KB 141. See para 2.13 above.

[13] [1983] 1 AC 410. See para 2.29 above.

(3) What should be the law where the defendant has negligently injured or imperilled someone other than the plaintiff, and the plaintiff, as a result, has foreseeably suffered a psychiatric illness?

(i) Should the reasonable foreseeability test be not only a necessary but also a sufficient test for the duty of care?

5.7 Some commentators and judges have argued that psychiatric illness (at least if shock-induced) should not be treated any differently from physical injury, and that no special or more restrictive rules ought to govern liability.[14] Mullany and Handford, for example, whilst conceding that *Alcock* has added a desirable degree of flexibility in some respects, believe that the law is still far too rigid and that a case by case approach, centred on reasonable foreseeability and without additional proximity requirements, would be preferable.[15] In this context it is argued that to make the existence of a duty of care turn solely on reasonable foreseeability rests on sound logic, that it would not necessarily open the floodgates, and that it would give the court greater flexibility to do justice and to deal with each individual case on its merits.

5.8 However, as Lord Bridge conceded in *McLoughlin*,[16] an important corollary of this flexibility is an element of uncertainty. To turn everything on reasonable foreseeability would open the way to a number of arguable claims which a more precisely fixed criterion of liability would exclude. Accordingly, one of the main effects of the adoption of this test would be to encourage claimants to litigate.[17] It is also arguable that a test of reasonable foreseeability would simply conceal underlying policy considerations which would continue to control the courts'

---

[14] See Lord Bridge in *McLoughlin v O'Brian* [1983] 1 AC 410, 441-443; Lord Wright in *Bourhill v Young* [1943] AC 92, 108; N J Mullany and P R Handford, *op cit*, esp pp 84, 310-312; B S Markesinis and S F Deakin, *Tort Law* (3rd ed 1994) p 121; A Watson, "Recovery for Nervous Shock: A Look at the Law and Some Thoughts of Reform" (1993) 12 Litigation 193, 198; S Hedley, "Hillsborough - Morbid Musings of a Reasonable Chief Constable" [1992] CLJ 16, 18; A Unger, "Undue Caution in the Lords" (1991) 141 NLJ 1729, 1730; J Williams, "Torts - Nervous Shock - Relation to Nominate Torts" (1968) Can BR 515, 516. On preliminary consultation this was also the view favoured by the Association of Personal Injury Lawyers.

[15] Mullany and Handford's thesis is supported by several reviewers of their book: see, eg, H Teff (1994) 10 PN 108; J Fleming (1994) Tort LR 202; N Solomon (1994) JPIL 169; S Todd (1993) 15 NZULR 466; B Hocking (1994) 1 Psychiatry, Psychology and Law 59. Of course, Mullany and Handford accept that where sound policy objections would rule out even physical injury claims (as, eg, in *Hill v Chief Constable of West Yorkshire* [1989] AC 53) no duty of care should be owed: see *op cit*, pp 84, 312. But following through the logic of their thesis they are driven to conclude that there ought to be liability even in variations of the standard secondary victim situation; eg where a wife suffers nervous shock as a consequence of concern for the legal position of her husband who has negligently injured a stranger; or where the plaintiff suffers nervous shock from the realisation that, had she been in a certain place at a certain time, she too would have been killed or injured by the negligent defendant : see *op cit*, 220-223. See also para 5.11 n 28 below.

[16] [1983] 1 AC 410, 442.

[17] See G Exall, "Nervous shock after Hillsborough" (1992) 136 SJ 13.

decision-making.[18] For example, under a foreseeability test there would be no separate requirement of direct perception. Cases of indirect perception, however, might nevertheless fail because the court might decide that the psychiatric illness was not foreseeable.

5.9   Moreover, it is at least arguable that the force of the reasonable foreseeability test as a determinant of the duty of care has been diminished since the demise of *Anns v Merton London Borough Council*.[19] In recent cases in which the House of Lords has examined the test for the existence of a duty of care in negligence it has made it clear - perhaps in response to the fear that policy arguments of the type considered in Part IV would otherwise be overlooked - that, in addition to reasonable foreseeability, a relationship of *proximity* must be established.[20] Moreover, in so far as different from proximity, the plaintiff must also show that it is just and reasonable to impose a duty of care. Where physical injury or damage is in issue, the existence of a nexus between the parties does not often give rise to any difficulty, and there is rarely any need to look beyond the foreseeability of the harm to determine whether an appropriate relationship of proximity between the parties exists.[21] If physical injury is inflicted to the person or property of another it always needs to be justified.[22] In the case of other kinds of damage, such as pure economic loss or mental injury, however, such proximity is not self-evident and there are policy arguments for restricting liability which need to be considered.

5.10   The approach of the House of Lords in *Alcock*, in which it was emphasised that in cases of negligently inflicted psychiatric illness proximity is a substantive and independent requirement, which has to be satisfied in addition to the test of

---

[18]   See generally, J Fleming, "Remoteness and Duty: The Control Devices in Liability for Negligence" (1953) 31 Can BR 471; J Steele, "Scepticism and the Law of Negligence" [1993] CLJ 437, 447-450; P G Heffey, "The Negligent Infliction of Nervous Shock in Road and Industrial Accidents: Part I" (1974) 48 ALJ 196, 199; H Teff, "The Hillsborough Football Disaster and Claims for 'Nervous Shock'" (1992) 32 Med Sci Law 251, 252-253; K J Nasir, "Nervous Shock and *Alcock*: The Judicial Buck Stops Here" (1992) 55 MLR 705, 707-708.

[19]   [1978] AC 728. Lord Wilberforce in *Anns* proposed a two stage test for establishing the existence of a duty of care, the first limb of which was subsequently interpreted as equating proximity with foreseeability in such a way that a prima facie duty arose where foreseeability alone was established. The second stage required the consideration of factors which might negative, reduce or limit the prima facie duty.

[20]   *Caparo Industries Plc v Dickman* [1990] 2 AC 605; *Murphy v Brentwood District Council* [1991] 1 AC 398.

[21]   See, for example, Lord Oliver in *Murphy v Brentwood District Council* [1991] 1 AC 398, 486-487. Cf *Marc Rich & Co AG v Bishop Rock Marine Co Ltd* [1994] 1 WLR 1071 (CA) (even though negligence resulted in physical damage to the plaintiff's person or property, not only must the damage have been reasonably foreseeable, but there must have been a relationship of proximity between the parties such that in all the circumstances it was fair, just and reasonable to impose a duty of care).

[22]   *Murphy v Brentwood District Council* [1991] 1 AC 398, 487.

reasonable foreseeability, is therefore consistent with the general approach of the courts to questions concerned with the existence of a duty of care.

5.11 Perhaps most importantly of all, if reasonable foreseeability were adopted as the sole determinant of the existence of a duty of care, the likely consequence would be a considerable expansion of the scope of liability.[23] This has certainly been the goal of those who champion such a test. And unless one simply uses the test to justify results which are in reality based on other policy factors, it would seem clear that the adoption of such a test must extend liability, because it is surely reasonably foreseeable that all manner of plaintiffs of reasonable fortitude may suffer psychiatric illness as a consequence of injury to, or fear for, a primary victim. While such width would naturally sweep up all deserving cases, it would do so not only at the expense of allowing more doubtful claims, but also at the risk of opening up the floodgates of litigation. The floodgates objection,[24] in its major sense of preventing a mass of claims from a single event, appears to be the primary explanation for the courts' caution in this sphere and it seems to us to have force in the context of psychiatric illness suffered by secondary victims. One thinks, for example, of all those who may foreseeably suffer psychiatric illness from watching a particularly gruesome news broadcast or from being present at a disaster at a sports event. Although it is true that in advance of seeing the consequences of implementing a less restrictive legal regime, the case for fearing the opening of the floodgates rests more on intuition and experience than on definitive proof,[25] we believe that the medical literature and surveys do provide some backing for the view that the floodgates would be opened if a psychiatric illness could sustain a negligence action in the same way that a physical injury can.[26] This conclusion is also supported by several reviewers of Mullany and Handford's book, *Tort Liability for Psychiatric Damage*. For example Tony Weir writes, "In cases of shock... if we go by foreseeability alone we are in for a large increase in litigation - expensive for the defendant if, as in physical injury cases, we virtually presume that the harm was foreseeable if it occurs as a result of unduly dangerous conduct...."[27] Professor Stanton is of the view that, "[A]n

---

[23] See K J Nasir, "Nervous Shock and *Alcock*: The Judicial Buck Stops Here" (1992) 55 MLR 705, 708. See also para 2.20 above. Lord Bridge, who advocated such an approach in *McLoughlin v O'Brian*, would have gone much further than previous law permitted and allowed recovery for nervous shock caused by the communication of bad news by a third party [1983] 1 AC 410, 442.

[24] See paras 4.2-4.6 above.

[25] See *Attia v British Gas Plc* [1988] 1 QB 304, 320, *per* Bingham LJ. On preliminary consultation we spoke to an economist and representatives of the insurance industry, amongst others, as to the "cost" of extending liability for psychiatric illness. The unanimous view was that nothing more than an unreliable "guesstimate" could be given. In particular, the effect of increased public awareness of the possibility of such claims is very hard to quantify.

[26] See para. 3.15 above. Although note the point there made that most of the surveys do not deal with secondary victims.

[27] [1993] CLJ 520, 521.

untrammelled foreseeability test is liable to produce chaos and 'control factors', with the inevitable anomalies they produce on the borderlines, are possibly the better of two evils."[28] In response to the argument that the cost, stress and strain of legal proceedings stop the opening of the floodgates, Loane Skene writes, "[O]ne might ask whether the traditional reluctance of plaintiffs to sue in such cases would continue if there were a surge of successful claims attracting widespread publicity".[29]

5.12 **We have provisionally concluded that special limitations over and above reasonable foreseeability should continue to be applied to claims for psychiatric illness where the defendant has negligently injured or imperilled someone other than the plaintiff and the plaintiff, as a result, has suffered a psychiatric illness. We ask consultees whether they agree with this provisional view. If they do not agree, please would they give their reasons.**

(ii) In applying the reasonable foreseeability test, should the plaintiff be assumed to be a person of reasonable fortitude?

5.13 Unless the defendant has prior knowledge of the plaintiff's susceptibility, the present law rules out claims for psychiatric illness by the abnormally sensitive in situations where a person of reasonable fortitude would not have suffered psychiatric illness.[30] It is not entirely clear to us whether this represents a more restrictive approach than is applied to other cases of personal injury. In *Haley v London Electricity Board*,[31] for example, a blind plaintiff recovered damages in negligence against the defendants when he tripped over a long-handled hammer left by them to fence a trench they had dug in the pavement. The obstacle was not a danger to sighted people. Nevertheless, given the number of blind people, it was held that the defendants should have reasonably foreseen that the plaintiff might be injured and, accordingly, should have taken different measures to fence the trench. By analogy, one might imagine that a defendant in most situations ought reasonably to foresee that there is a sufficiently high likelihood of there being abnormally sensitive "secondary victims" of his negligent conduct. If so, the present assumption that the plaintiff is a person of reasonable fortitude represents a restriction special to the realm of

---

[28] (1994) 23 Anglo-Am LR 249, 250. See also, eg D Robertson, "Liability in Negligence for Nervous Shock" (1994) 57 MLR 649, 660-662; R Bagshaw (1993) 109 LQR 691. Note that Mullany and Handford's thesis extends beyond the secondary victim cases so that, on the face of it, they would be suggesting a liability where, for example, a bank manager's negligent advice results in pecuniary loss and consequent psychiatric illness to the plaintiff, or where the DSS negligently refuses a benefit to a plaintiff who suffers psychiatric illness as a result: see the book review by Lunney (1993) Med LR 408, 411.

[29] (1994) Tort LJ 96, 99. See, similarly, J Stapleton, "In Restraint of Tort" in P Birks (ed), *The Frontiers of Liability* (1994) vol 2, p 95: "[T]he real root of concern may be that appellate courts suspect, and with reason it seems to me, that once a general duty to avoid nervous shock was recognised, many more individuals would be recognised as presenting the relevant symptoms to their GPs."

[30] See para 2.10 above.

[31] [1965] AC 778.

psychiatric illness. We are also concerned as to whether the distinction between reasonable fortitude and abnormal sensitivity is too crude, given that the temperaments of individuals differ widely. **We ask consultees: (a) whether they regard the emphasis on the plaintiff's reasonable fortitude as a restriction special to claims for psychiatric illness or, on the contrary, as no more than an application in the realm of psychiatric illness of the standard approach to reasonable foreseeability in personal injury cases; (b) whether in applying the reasonable foreseeability test, the law should continue to assume that the plaintiff is a person of reasonable fortitude or, on the contrary, whether they consider it unsatisfactory to distinguish between reasonable fortitude and abnormal sensitivity.**

(iii) Is any change required in relation to the establishing of a close tie of love and affection between the plaintiff and the primary victim?

5.14   We have seen[32] that the House of Lords in *Alcock* adopted a flexible approach to the necessary relationship between the plaintiff and the primary victim, eschewing any restriction to those with a particular blood or marital tie. What counts, their Lordships held, is the quality of the relationship, ie whether a close tie of love and affection existed. While such a tie may be rebuttably presumed in the case of parents, children and spouses and possibly fiancé(e)s, in other cases (ie in the cases of more distant relatives and friends) it must be proved by the plaintiff.

5.15   This emphasis on the quality of the relationship - the close tie of love and affection - has the great merit of enabling there to be recovery by those (eg close friends) who, arguably, have claims that are as meritorious as those of close members of the primary victim's family. However, this flexibility is gained at the expense of certainty, and a different approach would be to draw up a fixed list of qualifying relationships. Such a list would also have the advantage of avoiding altogether what may be embarrassing enquiries into the quality of a particular relationship. Furthermore, it would produce a measure of consistency with the Fatal Accidents Act 1976, which analogously deals with claims by "secondary victims", and does so by means of a fixed list.[33]

5.16   Another possibility for reform would be to build on the present approach by extending the list of relationships which raise a rebuttable presumption of a close tie of love and affection, while also allowing a plaintiff not on that list to prove a close tie of love and affection. This would give a measure of certainty, while retaining flexibility. Alternatively, one might have such a rebuttable list of

---

[32]   See paras 2.20-2.22 above.

[33]   We have now started work on preparing a consultation paper on the Fatal Accidents Act 1976. There are interesting differences between the approach to secondary victims under the 1976 Act and the approach to secondary victims who suffer psychiatric illness. For example, under the 1976 Act no duty of care to the dependants needs to be established and, for bereavement damages, no harm need be proved.

relationships, while *not* allowing a plaintiff outside that list to prove a close tie of love and affection. However, as against a system under which a plaintiff must prove on the facts of each case a close tie of love and affection, it is unclear to us whether such a list would minimise or, on the contrary, encourage potentially distressing and embarrassing enquiries into the quality of a relationship. At first blush it might be thought that a presumption would tend to obviate the need for such enquiries. As against that, it may be argued that, if it is for the plaintiff always to prove the close tie of love and affection, this minimises the incentive for defendants to produce evidence (most obviously, the report of a private investigator) so as to rebut the presumption.

5.17 **We ask consultees whether there should be: (a) a fixed list of qualifying relationships of close love and affection; or (b) a list of relationships in which there is a rebuttable presumption of a close tie of love and affection, while also allowing a plaintiff not on that list to prove a close tie of love and affection; or (c) a list of relationships in which there is a rebuttable presumption of a close tie of love and affection, while not allowing a plaintiff outside that list to prove a close tie of love and affection; or (d) no list at all, so that a plaintiff has to prove on the facts of each case a close tie of love and affection; or (e) an approach different to any of (a) to (d) for establishing a close tie of love and affection between the plaintiff and the primary victim?**

5.18 If it is thought that there should be a list of relationships of close love and affection (whether fixed or rebuttable), who should be on that list? The present rebuttable list covers parents, children and spouses. One might extend the list to include siblings (so that members of the primary victim's *nuclear family* are included).[34] More radically, one might draw on the wide list of "dependants" contained in section 1 of the Fatal Accidents Act 1976, which determines who is entitled to claim damages for loss of dependency under that Act. By section 1(3) "dependant" means wife, husband, child, grandchild, father, mother, grandparent, brother, sister, uncle, aunt or (as regards the last four) their issue, or, as inserted by the Administration of Justice Act 1982, ascendant beyond grandparent, descendant beyond grandchild, former husband or wife, person treated by the deceased as a child of the family or parent, or person living with the deceased as husband or wife immediately prior to the death and for at least two years before. Under section 1(5) the above list includes in-laws, half-brothers and sisters, and step-children. In contrast, by reason of section 1A(2), damages for bereavement can be claimed only by the spouse of the deceased and, where the deceased was a minor who was never married, by his parents if he was legitimate and by his mother if he was illegitimate. It should also be noted that even the wide list under section 1(3) excludes those living in a stable homosexual relationship.

---

[34] See Hidden J's comments in *Alcock* [1992] 1 AC 310, 337-338.

5.19   **If there is to be a list of relationships of close love and affection (whether fixed or rebuttable) our provisional view is that such a list should extend beyond parents, children and spouses, to include, at least, brothers and sisters and, also, to reflect the increased incidence of cohabitation between unmarried partners, it should include de facto spouses (defined using the wording in the Fatal Accidents Act 1976)[35] and those in a stable homosexual relationship.[36] By analogy to the Fatal Accidents Act, "child" or "parent" should include a person treated by the primary victim as a child of the family or parent.[37] We ask consultees whether they agree with this provisional proposal; and whether they have any other suggestions to make as to the content of such a list.**

5.20   If there is to be no fixed list of qualifying relationships, the question arises as to the content of the proof of a close tie of love and affection: if there is a list of relationships where the presumption is rebuttable, this question will arise only in relation to claims by those not on the list or to attempts by defendants to rebut the presumption. In *Alcock* Lord Ackner said that the tie of love and affection must be comparable to that normally existing between a spouse, parent, or child of the primary victim and the primary victim.[38] We do not interpret this dictum as ruling out a claim by, for example, a close friend of the primary victim.[39] **But our provisional view is that it is sufficient simply to say that a plaintiff must prove a close tie of love and affection to the primary victim. We ask consultees whether they agree with this provisional view. If they do not agree, what do they suggest instead?**

(iv) Should the requirements of closeness in time and space, and of perception through one's own unaided senses, be abandoned where there is a close tie of love and affection between the plaintiff and the primary victim?

5.21   After *Alcock* a plaintiff who establishes (a) a close tie of love and affection to the primary victim and (b) that he or she has suffered a foreseeable shock-induced psychiatric illness, will still be unable to recover damages unless he or she can also establish the two further requirements of (c) closeness in time and space to the accident and (d) perception through his or her own unaided senses.

---

[35]   Ie: "person living with the [primary victim] as husband or wife immediately prior to the [accident] and for at least two years before".

[36]   A possible definition could be "person living with the primary victim in a homosexual relationship immediately prior to the accident and for at least two years before".

[37]   This would cover stepchildren and stepparents and the offspring of cohabitees.

[38]   See para. 2.22 above.

[39]   The decision of the Outer House to deny damages in the Scottish case of *Robertson v Forth Road Bridge Joint Board (No 2)* 1994 SLT 568 is controversial as regards one of the two pursuers who, while a close friend of the primary victim, was held not to have a sufficiently close tie of love and affection to him: see Appendix, paras 2-3 below.

5.22   Hence in *Alcock* itself, Mr and Mrs Copoc,[40] whose son was killed, failed in their claims because, even though they clearly had a close tie of love and affection to the primary victim, they had not been present at Hillsborough. They had merely seen the general tragedy unfold on television and Mr Copoc had identified his son's body the following morning after having already been informed that he was dead. Again, in the light of *Alcock*, the first instance decision in *Ravenscroft v Rederiaktiebølaget Transatlantic*,[41] in which the court awarded a mother damages for psychiatric illness brought about by learning from others of the death of her son, was reversed on appeal.[42] The widow in *Taylor v Somerset Health Authority*[43] also failed because she could not bring her claim within the "immediate aftermath" extension of spatial and temporal proximity.

5.23   It can be strongly argued that all these decisions are unnecessarily restrictive. Once the range of claimants has been limited to those with a close tie of love and affection to the victim (and given that, according to the present law, the foreseeable psychiatric illness must have been shock-induced), it would appear that the central floodgates objection no longer has force. For the law to distinguish the claims for shock-induced psychiatric illness of one mother present at the scene of her son's death or at its immediate aftermath, from that of another mother who was not present at the scene but came across the aftermath several hours later or who heard about the accident from a friend or saw it on television,[44] might justly give rise to accusations of arbitrary and insensitive line-drawing.

5.24   Support for the abandonment of these two additional requirements where there is a close tie of love and affection to the primary victim may also be found in Deane J's judgment in *Jaensch v Coffey*. He said, "[T]he most important explanation of nervous shock resulting from injury to another is the existence of a close, constructive and loving relationship with that person (a 'close relative'), and ... it is largely immaterial whether the close relative is at the scene of the accident or how he or she learns of it."[45] This is also the approach advocated by Professor Trindade. In his view, "[The additional] requirements are illogical and arbitrary and could well

---

[40]   See para 2.18 above.

[41]   [1991] 3 All ER 73. *Hevican v Ruane* [1991] 3 All ER 65, on similar facts, must also now be regarded as wrongly decided.

[42]   [1992] 2 All ER 470 (Note). See para 2.33 above.

[43]   [1993] PIQR P262. See para 2.31 above.

[44]   The Young Solicitors' Group, in a response to our Fifth Programme of Law Reform (1991) Law Com No 200, supports recovery for shock-induced psychiatric illness caused through watching live or news coverage on television where the plaintiff can show a close relationship with a victim and the victim (who need not have been individually identifiable) has actually suffered injury.

[45]   (1984) 155 CLR 549, 600. Note also that in Germany it is no bar that the psychiatric illness is brought about by news of the accident: see Appendix, para 47 below.

be dispensed with, at least in the case of those who have a close tie of relationship or of care with the person killed, injured or put in peril by the negligence of the defendant. There is no danger that the abandonment of these requirements will result in open-ended liability in cases of nervous shock as the requirement of a close tie will continue to ensure that that liability is confined."[46] The medical literature is also of central importance for it shows that, for those with a close tie to the primary victim, merely learning about unexpected death or injury is a triggering event for PTSD.[47]

5.25   Support may also be found in the legislation enacted in three Australian jurisdictions, namely New South Wales, the Australian Capital Territory and the Northern Territory[48] (albeit that we do not consider satisfactory the precise details of this legislation, in that, for example, it treats grandparents more favourably than children or siblings). The legislation permits parents (but defined to include grandparents) and spouses (defined to include, in New South Wales and the Northern Territory, de facto spouses) - but not children or siblings except, as at common law, where they are present at the accident - to recover damages for nervous shock sustained as a result of the death or injury or peril of another caused by the wrongful act of the defendant, even though the parent or spouse was outside the sight or hearing of the accident. As far as we have been able to ascertain, this legislation has in no sense opened the floodgates of litigation in those states. Our research in respect of New South Wales indicates that there have been no reported cases in which a court has awarded damages to a secondary victim under section 4(1) of the Law Reform (Miscellaneous Provisions) Act 1944 who would not have

---

[46] F A Trindade, "The Principles Governing the Recovery of Damages for Negligently Caused Nervous Shock" [1986] CLJ 476, 499. See also K J Nasir, "Nervous Shock and *Alcock*: The Judicial Buck Stops Here" (1992) 55 MLR 705, 707, 713; H Teff, "Liability for Negligently Inflicted Nervous Shock" (1983) 99 LQR 100. Teff points to medical opinion which supports the view that, in some circumstances, hearing of the loss of a loved one in an accident could prompt an even stronger reaction than seeing it, given the human mind's propensity for constructing an image of an event even more gruesome than the reality. See also A Unger, "Undue Caution in the Lords" (1991) 141 NLJ 1729. See further D J Leibson, "Recovery of Damages for Emotional Distress Caused by Physical Injury to Another" (1975-1976) 15 Journal of Family Law 163, 196, n 79; B S Markesinis and S F Deakin, *Tort Law* (3rd ed 1994) p 126. See also A Ritchie, "Damages for Psychiatric Injuries" (1994) 144 NLJ 1690 and (1995) 145 NLJ 64 who in effect favours a widening of the "immediate aftermath".

[47] DSM-IV, para 309.81, p 424. B Green, "Defining Trauma: Terminology and Generic Stressor Dimensions" (1990) 20 Journal of Applied Social Psychology 1632; B Green et al, "Levels of functional impairment following a civilian disaster: the Beverley Hills Supper Club fire" (1983) 51 Journal of Consulting and Clinical Psychology 573. Hearing about death was also positively correlated to the development of PTSD in A Amick et al (1989) and P Saigh (1989) cited in J March, "What Constitutes a Stressor? The 'Criterion A' Issue" in J Davidson and E Foa (eds), *Posttraumatic Stress Disorder: DSM-IV and Beyond* (1993) p 45. See paras 3.5, 3.7 and 3.8 above.

[48] See Appendix, para 16 below.

been entitled to damages at common law (because not present at the accident).[49] Moreover, in correspondence with the New South Wales Law Reform Commission we have been told that the Government Insurance Office of New South Wales has received very few claims under section 4(1) of the 1944 Act.[50]

5.26   In *McLoughlin* Lord Bridge gave two hypothetical examples of deserving cases which would fall outside the restrictive limits put forward by Lord Wilberforce.[51] One of them was "of a mother who knows that her husband and children are staying in a certain hotel. She reads in her morning newspaper that it has been the scene of a disastrous fire. She sees in the paper a photograph of unidentifiable victims trapped on the top floor waving for help from the windows. She learns shortly afterwards that all her family have perished. She suffers an acute psychiatric illness."[52] It should be noted that if the additional proximity requirements were abandoned in cases where there is a close tie of love and affection to the primary victim, such a mother would be entitled to recover damages.[53]

5.27   **It is our provisional view that, for the above reasons, the requirements of closeness in time and space, and perception through one's own unaided senses, should be abandoned where there is a close tie of love and affection between the plaintiff and the primary victim. We ask consultees whether they agree. If consultees disagree with this provisional view, we ask: (a) do they disagree because they fear that an abandonment of those two requirements would open the floodgates of litigation and, if so, do they have any evidence to support their fears?; and (b) would they propose any changes to the present requirements of closeness in time and space and**

---

[49]   This is not to deny that there have been reported cases in which the extended entitlement to damages under s 4(1) of the 1944 Act has been relevant to other claims. Eg in *Smee v Tibbetts* (1953) 53 SR (NSW) 391 and in *State Rail Authority of New South Wales v Sharp* [1981] 1 NSWLR 240 the actual issue concerned a husband's claim for loss of consortium, which turned on whether a claim by his wife for psychiatric illness, on being informed of her daughter's death in an accident, was a claim for an actionable wrong. Liability under the 1944 Act to both the wife and the husband in *Sharp*, and to the wife in *Tibbetts*, was admitted. See Appendix, para 17.

[50]   In a letter to us dated 17 January 1995 the New South Wales Law Reform Commission write, "It is safe to assert that the 1944 Act has not led to an opening of the floodgates in NSW as far as claims for psychiatric illness are concerned". We would like to thank the Commission for its help on this matter.

[51]   See paras 2.16-2.17 above.

[52]   [1983] 1 AC 410, 442. For the other hypothetical example given by Lord Bridge, see para 2.24 n 79 above.

[53]   So would the husband in the example given by Trindade ("The Principles Governing the Recovery of Damages for Negligently Caused Nervous Shock" [1986] CLJ 476, 479) of a husband who is unable to have a sudden sensory perception of an accident to his wife because of his own bedridden condition but who suffers psychiatric illness when given a vivid and accurate description of the accident by a third party. It should also be noted that the controversial decision in *Schneider v Eisovitch* [1960] 2 QB 430, see paras 2.34-2.35 above, would be non-problematic under our provisional proposal.

perception through one's own unaided senses where there is a close tie of love and affection between the plaintiff and the primary victim? (Eg, should perception through live television qualify even if being told about the accident by a third party would not qualify?)

5.28   We should stress that in making our provisional proposal we have assumed that it will still be necessary to establish that a psychiatric illness to the plaintiff was foreseeable, ie that the defendant owed the plaintiff a duty of care. **But we also ask consultees whether they support the different approach taken in the Australian statutes[54] of allowing plaintiffs within certain degrees of relationship to claim without having to establish that he or she is owed a duty of care.**

(v) Should those who cannot establish a close tie of love and affection to the primary victim be able to recover? If so, in what circumstances?

(a) Bystanders

5.29   In addition to the established categories of the rescuer and involuntary participant, the House of Lords in *Alcock* refused to rule out completely recovery by mere "bystanders". However, the Court of Appeal in *McFarlane v EE Caledonia Ltd*[55] rejected their Lordships' dicta and did rule out such claims.[56] We believe that there would be a serious danger of opening the floodgates of litigation if bystanders were able to recover damages for psychiatric illness simply on the basis of the reasonable foreseeability test. For example, a whole range of strangers of reasonable fortitude may potentially suffer a shock-induced psychiatric illness from the depiction of tragic events, like Hillsborough, on television. Although it may be true that strangers are less prone to shock-induced psychiatric illness than those who are emotionally attached to primary victims, it is hard to discount such illness as not reasonably foreseeable.

5.30   In our view, therefore, the central issue is whether bystanders should ever be able to recover and, if they can, what restrictions should apply. Three main possible answers may be suggested. First, that the conclusion of the Court of Appeal in *McFarlane v EE Caledonia Ltd* should be supported so that claims by bystanders should be ruled out in all circumstances. Secondly, that the dicta of Lords Keith and Oliver in *Alcock*[57] should be supported so that, assuming closeness in time and space to the accident and perception through one's own unaided senses, there could

---

[54]   Appendix, para 17. A similar approach is taken to the recovery of economic loss and bereavement damages by dependants under the Fatal Accidents Act 1976 although, in contrast to the Australian statutes (see Appendix, para 18 below), the dependants under the 1976 Act must first show that the deceased had an actionable claim.

[55]   [1994] 2 All ER 1.

[56]   See para 2.24 above.

[57]   See para 2.24 above.

be recovery where the accident is particularly horrific. Or thirdly, one could insist that bystanders, who are close in time and space to the accident (including the immediate aftermath) and who perceive it through their own unaided senses, can recover. Although the second answer gains some support from the medical literature,[58] it has the disadvantage of leaving uncertain what constitutes a particularly horrific accident. Some might find it hard to see, for example, why the Hillsborough tragedy itself did not qualify as such an accident. As between the first and third answers, the dispute essentially turns on whether it is believed that the floodgates of litigation would be opened if claims by those bystanders who were close to the accident in time and space and who perceived the accident through their own unaided senses were to be allowed. On the one hand, the time and space and direct perception restrictions would mean that the class of bystanders able to claim would be restricted to some degree. But in some circumstances - for example, a tragedy at an air-show or a sporting event - the number of those bystanders might be huge. **We invite the views of consultees as to whether mere bystanders should be able to recover for shock-induced psychiatric illness and, if so, in what circumstances.**

(b) Rescuers

5.31 While there may be some uncertainty at the fringes in deciding whether a person is properly classified as a rescuer, rather than as a bystander,[59] we do not think it would be helpful to try to articulate more precisely what counts as a rescue for these purposes. It seems preferable to leave the courts with some discretion in deciding whether a particular intervenor deserves to recover damages for psychiatric illness in line with the overall policy of not discouraging rescue.

5.32 A further question is whether, in contrast to the position of ordinary rescuers, *professional* rescuers (for example, firemen and policemen) should be precluded from recovering damages for negligently inflicted psychiatric illness sustained in the course of carrying out their duties. The policy of not discouraging rescue is, arguably, inapplicable to such rescuers in that they have a legal duty to rescue. Moreover it may be thought that those who have chosen to take on such jobs have voluntarily accepted the risk of being exposed to horrifying events. Certainly the recent strong criticism in several newspapers[60] of the out-of-court settlements reached with police officers involved in rescue work at Hillsborough indicates that there is a widely-shared view that professionals should be expected to cope with shocking events and should not be treated sympathetically by the law if they are unable to do so.

---

[58] See para 3.9 above.

[59] See para 2.26 above.

[60] See, eg, the editorials "Moral blackmail" in the *Daily Telegraph* of 3 February 1995 and "Stress on the beat" in *The Times* of 4 February 1995.

5.33   On the other hand, it is well-established that a professional rescuer can recover for physical injuries sustained in the course of a rescue,[61] and it is not easy to see how one can justify a different approach for psychiatric illness as opposed to physical injury. It may also be thought invidious to distinguish between the claims for psychiatric illness of a fireman or policeman who is off duty and carries out a rescue and the fireman or policeman who carries out a rescue while on duty. Moreover the effect of disallowing claims for physical injury or psychiatric illness might be to discourage professional rescuers from pushing themselves beyond their minimum legal obligations. And while it is plainly true that a professional accepts that he or she will be faced with dangerous or shocking situations, this does not mean that he or she has chosen to give up a legal entitlement to recover damages for injury or illness *where that danger or horror has been brought about by another's wrong.*

5.34   If one believes that professional rescuers should not be precluded from recovering damages for psychiatric illness, it may still be argued that they should only be able to recover where it was reasonably foreseeable that even a hardened professional would suffer a psychiatric illness. That is, the usual approach of the plaintiff being assumed to be a person of reasonable fortitude[62] might be modified by expecting a professional "to be particularly thick-skinned when confronted with gruesome sights..."[63] It should also be noted that, even if the relevant legal principles are the same for professional and ordinary rescuers, the former will in practice often face greater difficulties in establishing liability than the latter: for example, as he or she is exposed to many shocking events, a professional rescuer will often have difficulty establishing that the particular event *caused* the psychiatric illness.[64]

5.35   **We ask consultees whether they agree with our provisional view that it would be unhelpful to lay down in legislation a definition of what counts as a rescue. We also invite the views of consultees as to whether professional rescuers should be precluded from recovering damages for negligently inflicted psychiatric illness sustained in the course of carrying out their duties; and, if not so precluded, we ask for views as to whether the same legal principles should be applied to determine the recovery of damages for negligently inflicted psychiatric illness by professional rescuers as are applied to ordinary rescuers.**

[61]   See para 2.27 above.

[62]   See para 2.10 above.

[63]   M Jones, *Textbook on Torts* (4th ed 1993) p 103.

[64]   See para 3.6 n 29.

(c) Involuntary participants

5.36 According to Lord Oliver in *Alcock*,[65] the type of case here in issue is "where the negligent act of the defendant has put the plaintiff in the position of being, or thinking that he is about to be or has been the involuntary cause of another's death or injury, and the illness complained of stems from the shock to the plaintiff of the consciousness of this supposed fact." Lord Oliver went on to say, "The fact that the defendant's negligent conduct has foreseeably put the plaintiff in the position of being an unwilling participant in the event establishes of itself a sufficiently proximate relationship between them, and the principal question is whether, in the circumstances, injury of that type to that plaintiff was or was not reasonably foreseeable."

5.37 We consider this to be a helpful approach.[66] But it should be noted that, in contrast to the facts of *Dooley v Cammell Laird Co Ltd*,[67] Lord Oliver's formulation, on the face of it, would allow an involuntary participant to recover even though the shock was not experienced through his or her own unaided senses and even though he or she was not close to the accident in time and space. For example, it would cover the case of a signalman who, by reason of operating his employer's faulty equipment, reasonably believes that he has been instrumental in causing a train crash (out of sight or hearing) and suffers a shock-induced psychiatric illness as a consequence. We believe that a signalman in that situation probably ought to be able to recover damages as there is no floodgates objection. We therefore do not regard Lord Oliver's formulation as being too wide-ranging. **Our provisional view is that there ought to be a special rule, as set out by Lord Oliver in *Alcock*, applicable to involuntary participants. Do consultees agree? If they do not agree, please would they give their reasons.**

(vi) Should one abandon the requirement (in secondary victim cases) that the psychiatric illness must have been shock-induced?

5.38 As we have seen,[68] it is clear law after *Alcock* that in secondary victim cases the psychiatric illness must have been shock-induced if it is to be compensatable. This rule has been criticised as artificial and unfair.[69] In the words of Mullany and

---

[65] [1992] 1 AC 310, 408. See para 2.28 above.

[66] The inclusion of involuntary participants within the class of permissible claimants would appear justified in medical terms: see B Green, "Defining Trauma: Terminology and Generic Stressor Dimensions" (1990) 20 Journal of Applied Social Psychology 1632, 1638.

[67] [1951] 1 Lloyd's Rep 271. See para 2.28 above.

[68] See paras 2.5 and 2.7 above.

[69] F A Trindade, "The Principles Governing the Recovery of Damages for Negligently Caused Nervous Shock" [1986] CLJ 476, 478-480; H Teff, "The Hillsborough Football Disaster and Claims for 'Nervous Shock'" (1992) 32 Med Sci Law 251, 253. See also S Todd, "Duties of Care: The New Zealand Jurisprudence Part 1: General Principles of Duty" (1993) 9 PN 2, 6; N Grace, "Doctors, Damages and Nervous Shock" (1986) 2 PN

Handford, "Not only where psychiatric damage results from a gradual accrual of shock, but also where mental distress (which on one view rightly does not sound in damages) leads to or transmutes into recognisable psychiatric damage, that damage should be compensable. That it started life as grief, sorrow, worry or anger is not to the point. The unnecessary 'shock' requirement stems, no doubt, from the inaccurate and misleading language of this category of claim."[70] Certainly it can be strongly argued that the distinction between gradually sustained psychiatric illness and psychiatric illness caused by a sudden shock does not reflect the underlying merits of claims. Should one distinguish, for example, between (a) the mother who suffers psychiatric illness as a result of seeing, or hearing about, her son's sudden death and (b) the mother who suffers psychiatric illness as a result of watching her son slowly die in hospital and (c) the mother who suffers psychiatric illness from looking after her injured son? "The fact that one claimant's experience is less protracted than another's does not mean that the latter has suffered any the less - on the contrary, on an abstract analysis he or she will usually have suffered more".[71] The rule has also been described as anachronistic in so far as it originated in cases of nervous shock where the plaintiff was threatened with physical injury by a sudden impact.[72] There is also some confusion as to the suddenness required for shock: in *Alcock* itself Lord Oliver's speech, for example, can be read as suggesting that the claim in that case should be denied because the shock was gradual rather than sudden and even though the period of time before the plaintiffs discovered for certain the fate of their loved ones was in no case more than twenty hours. Abolition of the need for shock would also have the advantage of easing the difficulty when quantifying damages of separating out the effects of a shock-induced psychiatric illness from a non-shock-induced psychiatric illness that would have been suffered in any event.[73]

5.39   On the other hand, the requirement of shock does operate to cut down substantially the range of potential plaintiffs. To allow recovery for psychiatric illness resulting from subsequent contact with the victim would involve a large extension of the

46, 49; B S Markesinis and S F Deakin *Tort Law* (3rd ed 1994) p 124; and J Swanton, "Issues in Tort Liability for Nervous Shock" (1992) 66 ALJ 495, 500.

[70] *Op cit*, p 206.

[71] K J Nasir, "Nervous Shock and *Alcock*: The Judicial Buck Stops Here" (1992) 55 MLR 705, 709.

[72] K J Nasir, "Nervous Shock and *Alcock*: The Judicial Buck Stops Here" (1992) 55 MLR 705, 709. The link is made by N Grace, "Doctors, Damages and Nervous Shock" (1985) 2 PN 46, 48-49. Recovery for gradually sustained injury has, of course, never been in doubt for physical injury. Common industrial injuries are often gradually sustained, or "non-traumatic". Examples of such physical injuries include dust diseases, asbestosis, repetitive movement injury, deafness and dermatitis. There are also product-caused injuries, such as adverse drug reactions, and environmental diseases including diseases caused by fertilisers: see generally J Stapleton, *Disease and the Compensation Debate* (1986).

[73] Para 2.8 above.

scope of liability.[74] It is also arguable that, without the element of shock, the risk of fraudulent claims would be significantly increased. Is there not a risk, for example, that nearly all those entitled to bring an action under the Fatal Accidents Act 1976 (for the wrongful death of another) would add a claim for psychiatric illness caused by the bereavement, and that it would be difficult for the courts to distinguish between the "ordinary" grief of bereavement[75] and a psychiatric illness consequent on bereavement? The question whether the psychiatric illness was *caused* by the accident might also be rendered more difficult if the shock requirement were removed.

5.40 **We invite the views of consultees as to whether the requirement, in secondary victim cases, that the psychiatric illness must have been shock-induced should be abandoned.**

(vii) Instead of, or in addition to, other restrictions, should it be a requirement that the psychiatric illness be of a particular severity?

5.41 In our forthcoming consultation paper on damages for non-pecuniary loss[76] we shall be considering the arguments for and against introducing a threshold of severity in respect of the assessment of damages for non-pecuniary loss in all personal injury cases. The question at issue here is rather, should a severity threshold be introduced *at the liability stage* in psychiatric illness cases?

5.42 It may be argued that one way of avoiding opening the floodgates of litigation and, more particularly, of restricting the risk of fraudulent and exaggerated claims, is to insist that the plaintiff must prove not only that he or she has been caused to suffer a recognisable psychiatric illness but also that the psychiatric illness has crossed a certain threshold of severity. In this respect it is interesting to note that under the controversial new criminal injuries compensation scheme,[77] personal injury for which compensation is payable includes "mental injury (that is, a medically recognised psychiatric or psychological illness) either resulting directly from ... physical injury or occurring without any physical injury."[78] Mental injury is then further defined as a "*disabling* mental disorder where the psychological and/or physical symptoms

---

[74] J Swanton, "Issues in Tort Liability for Nervous Shock", (1992) 66 ALJ 495, 499-500.

[75] For which damages of £7,500 are recoverable by the parents or spouse of the deceased under s 1A of the Act.

[76] See para 1.1, n 3 above.

[77] "Criminal Injuries Compensation - The Tariff Scheme" (1994)(available from the Criminal Injuries Compensation Authority): see also the guide published by the Criminal Injuries Compensation Authority, "Victims of Crimes of Violence: A Guide to Criminal Injuries Compensation (Issue No 1, March 1994). In *R v Secretary of State for the Home Department, ex p Fire Brigades Union* [1995] 2 WLR 1 the Court of Appeal decided, in judicial review proceedings, that the new scheme is invalid. There has been an appeal to the House of Lords.

[78] Note 1 to para 5 of the Tariff Scheme.

and disability persist for more than six weeks from the incident."[79] (emphasis added)

5.43 On the other hand, the very fact that a psychiatric illness is required for liability can in itself be regarded as constituting a severity requirement in that, in the absence of concomitant physical injury, it rules out liability for mere mental distress which has been negligently inflicted.[80] And while even the distinction between a psychiatric illness and mental distress is, arguably, a difference of degree and not kind, the fixing of acceptable criteria which would have to be satisfied for a psychiatric illness to be of sufficient severity would be difficult.

5.44 **Our provisional view is that damages for psychiatric illness should continue to be recoverable irrespective of whether the psychiatric illness is of a particular severity. Do consultees agree? If they do not agree, please would they give their reasons.**

(viii) Should recovery be barred where the primary victim is the defendant?

5.45 Say a person causes his daughter or a rescuer to suffer a shock-induced psychiatric illness by witnessing his attempt to commit suicide (eg by throwing himself from a building)? Or say a person is wholly responsible for a car accident in which she is killed, thereby causing her son or a rescuer to suffer a foreseeable shock-induced psychiatric illness? Assuming all other criteria for the recovery of damages for psychiatric illness in the tort of negligence are satisfied, should liability nevertheless be barred because the primary victim is the defendant (that is, because the defendant's injury is self-inflicted)?

---

[79] It is also interesting to note that it has been suggested that the minimum period of duration of symptoms which must elapse before a diagnosis of PTSD can be made should be increased from one month to three, implying a chronic disorder: B Rothbaum and E Foa, "Suggested Recommendations for DSM-IV: Duration, Subtypes, and Posttraumatic Stress Disorder In Relation to Adjustment Disorder" in J Davidson and E Foa (eds), *Posttraumatic Stress Disorder: DSM-IV and Beyond* (1993) Appendix 2, p 241. DSM-IV does indeed provide that the specifier "chronic" should be used when symptoms last 3 months or longer. However, it has also been suggested that the requirement for one-month duration should be dropped on the basis that there is no evidence that PTSD is to be regarded any less seriously for being brief: A Blank, "Suggested Recommendations for DSM-IV on Course and Sub-types" in Davidson and Foa (eds), *op cit*, Appendix 1, 237, 238. But see the new diagnostic category included in DSM-IV, Acute Stress Disorder, para 308.3, pp 429-432 and Appendix D, p 783: para 4.5 n 13 above.

[80] In *Aggravated, Exemplary and Restitutionary Damages* (1993) Consultation Paper No 132, paras 6.53 and 8.18, we asked consultees, in the context of aggravated damages, for their views as to whether compensatory damages for intangible loss should be available in respect of all wrongs or only some. Cf the law in France and in the United States: see Appendix, paras 44-45 and 42-43.

5.46 We have seen that, while there is no English authority directly in point, dicta suggest that, as in Australia, recovery will indeed be barred in this situation.[81] This also appears to be the law in, for example, Scotland,[82] Canada,[83] and Germany[84].

5.47 The principal argument in favour of such a restriction is that putting people under a duty to take care of their own life or limb, so as not to cause others to sustain psychiatric illness, places an undesirable and burdensome restriction on self-determination.[85] People ought to be free to injure or endanger themselves, subject only to the relatively minor restriction that, in doing so, they should not *physically* harm or endanger others. It can also be argued that it is somewhat distasteful for a person to be liable to those who have a close tie of love and affection for him or her. It may also be thought insensitive for the law to add to the woes of an injured primary victim - including, in an extreme case, a person who has been so unbalanced as to commit or attempt suicide - by allowing actions against him or her (or his or her estate) for the consequential psychiatric illness of others.

5.48 Some academic commentators[86] have, however, criticised this restriction primarily on the basis that, as psychiatric illness should be taken as seriously as physical injury or property damage, people ought to think about, and be answerable for, the psychiatric, as well as the physical, consequences to others of their actions. Certainly it is true that there would be no impediment to liability if physical injury or damage to property (or even psychiatric illness arising from a fear of physical injury to oneself) has been caused to the plaintiff by someone who has negligently or deliberately injured himself or herself (for example, where deliberately walking onto a railway line to kill oneself causes a train crash). Furthermore it is commonplace in road accident cases, where insurance is compulsory, for one member of a family to sue another; and, in practice, if the defendant is not insured, it is unlikely that a relative would sue.

---

[81] See paras 2.40-2.41 above.

[82] See Appendix, para 4.

[83] See Appendix, para 32.

[84] See Appendix, para 48.

[85] *Ibid.*

[86] See, eg, N J Mullany and P R Handford, *op cit*, pp 217-220; F A Trindade, "The Principles Governing the Recovery of Damages for Negligently Caused Nervous Shock" [1986] CLJ 476, 481-482; M Jones, *Textbook on Torts* (4th ed 1993) p 111. Mullany and Handford, *op cit*, at p 132, give the following vivid example from Lord Robertson's judgment in *Bourhill v Young* 1941 SC 395, 399: "[W]hy...should a window-cleaner (or his estate) who, due to his own negligence, falls from a height and impales himself upon spiked railings not be held liable for the shock-induced psychiatric harm caused to a pregnant woman who witnesses the incident from the window of her house on the opposite side of the street?".

5.49   Even if in general one is in favour of the bar, it is hard to dispute that it produces difficulty where the primary victim's negligence has contributed to an accident with another negligent party ("the tortfeasor"). For in that situation it seems unfair to the tortfeasor not to allow any right of contribution against the primary victim. Say, for example, D1 is a pedestrian who steps out into a road thereby causing D2, who is driving at an excessive speed, to crash into a wall injuring himself. P, D2's son, who witnesses the immediate aftermath of the accident, suffers a psychiatric illness. If D1 is 25% responsible for the accident, and D2 75% responsible, it would seem unfair if P could recover 100% damages from D1, while D1 has no right of contribution against D2 (because the bar to recovery for self-inflicted injury means that D2 commits no tort against P). As Lord Oliver said in *Alcock*, "I can visualise great difficulty arising ... where the accident, though not solely caused by the primary victim has been materially contributed to by his negligence. If, for instance, the primary victim is himself 75 per cent responsible for the accident, it would be a curious and wholly unfair situation if the plaintiff were enabled to recover damages for his or her traumatic injury from the person responsible only in a minor degree whilst he in turn remained unable to recover any contribution from the person primarily responsible since the latter's negligence vis-a-vis the plaintiff would not even have been tortious."[87]

5.50   This difficulty constitutes a further argument for wholly rejecting the bar to recovery where the primary victim is the defendant. But if one favours the bar, how can this particular difficulty be overcome? One possible solution, and the one applied in Germany,[88] is to reduce the plaintiff's damages in line with the contributory negligence of the primary victim. But this would contradict the underlying approach to claims for psychiatric illness in English law, whereby the secondary victim's claim rests on a duty of care owed to him or her and is not viewed as a derivative claim arising on a duty owed to the primary victim.[89] An alternative solution would therefore simply be to limit the scope of the bar by not applying it in respect of claims for contribution.

5.51   **We ask consultees (a) should there be a bar to the recovery of damages for psychiatric illness where the primary victim is the defendant?; and, if so, (b) what should be the solution to the difficulty relating to contribution articulated by Lord Oliver in *Alcock*?**

---

[87]   [1992] 1 AC 310, 418.

[88]   See Appendix, para 48 below.

[89]   Mullany and Handford, *op cit*, pp 251-256. See para 4.13 above. This contrasts with the approach under s 5 of the Fatal Accidents Act 1976.

(ix) Where the plaintiff suffers psychiatric illness from the communication of true news about a primary victim, when does the communication of the news break the chain of causation between the negligence of the defendant causing the injury to the primary victim and the psychiatric illness of the plaintiff?

5.52   If our proposal on question *(iv)* above were to be accepted, so that a person with a close tie of love and affection to the primary victim could recover damages for a shock-induced psychiatric illness where that shock has been brought about by a third party's communication or broadcast, the question would arise as to the circumstances in which communication or broadcasting of true news breaks the chain of causation between the negligence of the defendant causing the injury to the primary victim and the psychiatric illness of the plaintiff. There seems no reason to doubt that the normal principles of causation at common law would satisfactorily resolve this problem.[90]   Applying them, it would seem, for example, that unreasonable sensational reporting or television broadcasting that departs from the broadcasting code of ethics could break the chain of causation from the defendant's negligence. The court would no doubt be influenced by whether the plaintiff would have a cause of action against the communicator or broadcaster of the news.[91] **We are of the provisional view that the application of the normal principles of causation would satisfactorily answer this question. Do consultees agree with this provisional view? If they do not agree, please would they give their reasons.**

(4) What should be the law where the defendant has negligently damaged or imperilled property belonging to the plaintiff or to a third party and the plaintiff, as a result, has foreseeably suffered a psychiatric illness?

5.53   We have seen[92] that the law in this area is not clear, but that, in the light of *Attia v British Gas Plc*,[93] it appears that foreseeable psychiatric illness consequent on damage to, or fear for, property may be recoverable.[94] Our provisional view is that the Court of Appeal's judgment in *Attia* is persuasive and that there is no good reason to deny all liability for a psychiatric illness arising out of damage or danger to property.

---

[90]   Stocker LJ in the *Alcock* case considered that a broadcast containing substantial elements of editing and commentary constitutes a *novus actus interveniens* breaking the chain of causation: [1992] 1 AC 310, 380. For criticism of that suggestion see M Davie "Negligently Inflicted Psychiatric Illness: The Hillsborough Case in the House of Lords" (1992) 43 NILQ 237, 246 n 49.

[91]   See paras 5.57-5.58 below.

[92]   See paras 2.42-2.44 above.

[93]   [1988] QB 304.

[94]   In contrast, shock attributable to non-human interests is not covered by the Criminal Injuries Compensation Tariff Scheme.

5.54   As to the circumstances in which there should be such liability, it surely could not be right - where the property damaged or imperilled belongs to someone other than the plaintiff - for the law to be less restrictive than where the safety of, or injury to, another person is involved. Our provisional view, therefore, is that in such cases involving damage or danger to another person's property there should be additional criteria for establishing liability over and above the requirement that the incidence of psychiatric illness should be reasonably foreseeable; and that those criteria should be analogous to, and certainly no less restrictive than, those adopted where human safety or injury to another is involved. So one may wish to insist that: (a) the plaintiff can show a close attachment to the property (for example, by living in a house, even though the house is owned by someone else); (b) that he or she was present at the time of the damage; and (c) that he or she perceived the damage through his or her unaided senses rather than being told of it or seeing it on television. Indeed even if the law were to be reformed in accordance with our provisional view above[95] - so that a plaintiff with a close tie of love and affection to the primary victim would be able to recover irrespective of closeness to the accident in time and space and of perception through his or her own unaided senses - it might be appropriate to continue to require that in cases of damage or danger to another's property all three proximity elements are satisfied. One may also consider that, whatever the position where human safety or injury is involved, it should be a continued requirement that psychiatric illness consequent on damage or danger to another's property must have been shock-induced.

5.55   In contrast, it is less obvious that special restrictions should apply where the property damaged, or imperilled, belongs to the plaintiff. Here the plaintiff is a primary victim and, in line with cases where a plaintiff is physically injured or in personal danger, it is legitimate to take the view that no special restrictions should apply, so that psychiatric illness is simply compensatable where it is reasonably foreseeable. This proposition derives support from the tenor of the judgments of the Court of Appeal in *Attia v British Gas Plc*.[96] On the other hand, as we have commented above,[97] it might be thought odd if a plaintiff could recover more easily for psychiatric illness consequent on damage to his or her property (eg a house) than for psychiatric illness consequent on personal injury to another (eg his or her spouse).

5.56   **We ask consultees: (a) whether they agree with our provisional view that where psychiatric illness is consequent on damage, or danger, to the property of someone other than the plaintiff, criteria analogous to, but no less restrictive than, those applied where human safety or injury to another**

---

[95]   See para 5.27 above.

[96]   [1988] QB 304: see para 2.44 above.

[97]   See para 2.44 above.

is involved, should be insisted on; (b) whether in that situation (ie where the psychiatric illness arises from damage to, or fear for, property belonging to someone other than the plaintiff) they would be in favour of retaining all three proximity elements and also the requirement that the psychiatric illness must have been shock-induced; (c) whether they consider that psychiatric illness consequent on damage, or danger, to one's own property should be equated with psychiatric illness consequent on personal injury, or danger, to oneself so that no special restrictions, over and above reasonable foreseeability, should be applied, and if not what they consider the special restrictions should be.

(5) Should there be liability for the negligent communication of news to the plaintiff foreseeably causing him or her to suffer a psychiatric illness?

5.57 There appears to be no absolute rule under English law militating against the recognition of a duty of care in relation to the communication of news, although the indications are that there is no such liability, especially where news is in fact true.[98] Mullany and Handford argue that the liability of conveyers of news ought not to be limited "by the introduction of the same sorts of arbitrary restrictions that have thwarted the sensible development of other aspects of the law governing psychiatric damage" and that liability should simply depend on whether (shock-induced) psychiatric illness was foreseeable.[99] On this test, the truth or falsity of the information conveyed would be irrelevant. Most other commentators, however, express the need for caution, at least as regards statements which are true.[100]

5.58 The recognition of a duty to take care not to cause psychiatric illness by the style or manner in which one delivers shocking news which is *true*, may be thought to involve a more oppressive fetter on communicators than would the recognition of a duty to take care not to put into circulation shocking news which is false. Further, the psychiatric illness of the person to whom the true news is given will often also be attributable to the nature of the news itself: hence it may be extremely difficult to establish whether and to what extent a plaintiff's psychiatric illness is due to the shock of the news itself or to the way in which it was conveyed.[101] It is arguable, however, that this difficulty is a problem of causation alone and that it should not in itself prevent a duty of care arising. Where the true news concerns someone other than the plaintiff, there is also a legitimate fear that the floodgates of litigation would be opened if a duty of care was imposed, although this objection could be met by

---

[98] See paras 2.45-2.48 above.

[99] N J Mullany & P R Handford, *Tort Liability for Psychiatric Damage* (1993) p 191.

[100] Eg B S Markesinis & S F Deakin, *Tort Law* (3rd ed 1994) pp 127-128; and reviews of Mullany and Handford's book by H Teff (1994) 10 PN 108; M Lunney (1993) 1 Med L Rev 408, 411; S Todd (1993) 15 NZULR 466, 468.

[101] See B S Markesinis & S F Deakin, *Tort Law* (3rd ed 1994) p 127; S Todd (1993) 15 NZULR 466, 468.

restricting claims to those with a close tie of love and affection to the person injured or imperilled. Perhaps the most powerful argument against permitting plaintiffs to sue those who deliver true bad news carelessly is that this would place an undesirable burden on those whose duty it is to deliver distressing news. The police, the medical profession and social workers, for example, often have to deliver distressing news, and it is said that the utility of subjecting them to a duty of care is not self evident.[102] Indeed, the recognition of a duty to communicate true bad news carefully might lead to less than full and frank disclosure of details. Moreover, in the case of the media - which conveys information because it is newsworthy or in order to inform the public of matters (including disasters) which are of general interest - a duty to report true news carefully would arguably raise problems concerned with the infringement of freedom of speech, under Article 10 of the European Convention of Human Rights; and the creation of such a duty might also tend to devalue the countervailing interest of the public at large in receiving the information in question.[103] On the other hand, it can be argued that a duty to break bad news gently might discourage the worst kind of sensational reporting by the press. It would also impose standards upon the media regarding the specificity of the information which it conveys.[104] Against this, other mechanisms already exist for ensuring that standards are observed regarding the manner and style of both media communications and communications by those who may have to convey bad news as part of their official duties.[105]

5.59   Some of the above arguments, such as the countervailing interest in freedom of communication and in free speech, apply also, although with less weight, when we turn to consider questions of liability arising from *false* statements which are made negligently. A duty to check the truth of statements which might give rise to shock-induced psychiatric injury could also inhibit promptness and lead to undesirable delay in communicating news. This may be a particularly important consideration from the perspective of the press and broadcast media, where speedy reporting is highly valued by the public. On the other hand, the arguments against a duty of care seem far less compelling where the information is false: potential liability would encourage those who communicate information to check its veracity. A duty of care

---

[102] M Lunney [1993] Med L Rev 408, 411. H Teff (1994) 10 PN 108 also warns that harsh consequences could follow if conveyers of true bad news are held liable by applying mechanically a test of foreseeability and without taking adequate account of how difficult it can be to break as well as to receive bad news.

[103] B S Markesinis & S F Deakin, *Tort Law* (3rd ed 1994) p 128.

[104] For example, where, very soon after a disaster, it is reported on radio or TV that the disaster has occurred and that it is already known that Mr X, Mrs Y and Z's child are among those definitely killed. F Trindade & P Cane, *The Law of Torts in Australia* (2nd ed 1993) p 347 express the view that "[u]sually, no doubt, the media could not be sued for reporting bad news, provided they reasonably believed it to be true. But ... it might be thought that the media should be under a legal duty to stay quiet until relatives have been informed."

[105] One example is the broadcasting code of ethics (referred to in *Alcock* [1992] 1 AC 310).

is owed in certain circumstances under English law in respect of negligent statements which cause economic loss,[106] and it might be argued with some force that economic injury should not be accorded any better protection than injury which is psychiatric in nature.

5.60 **We ask consultees whether there should be liability for the negligent communication of news to the plaintiff causing him or her a foreseeable psychiatric illness. In particular we ask: (a) do consultees agree with our provisional view that the existence of a duty of care should not rest on foreseeability alone?; (b) if there are circumstances in which liability should be imposed, what are those circumstances?; (c) should a distinction be drawn depending on whether the news conveyed is true or false?; (d) should a further distinction be drawn between communication by the media to the public at large (although the information itself may specifically affect the plaintiff) and communication by officials and other individuals to specific individuals?**

(6) Should there be liability where an employer has negligently overburdened its employee with work thereby foreseeably causing him or her to suffer a psychiatric illness?

5.61 We have already mentioned the landmark decision in *Walker v Northumberland CC*,[107] in which a social worker was awarded damages for psychiatric illness caused by stress at work; and we have also observed[108] that there are other miscellaneous instances[109] in which a primary victim is probably entitled to damages for negligently inflicted psychiatric illness. The essential feature of these cases is that, because the plaintiff is the primary victim, there is no problem about opening the floodgates of litigation in its primary sense of opening the way for an indeterminate number of claims from a single breach of duty. Indeed it is noteworthy in this regard that Mr Walker was also held entitled to recover for breach of his employer's contractual duty of care; and, so far as we are aware, no special restrictions have been imposed on liability for psychiatric illness in contract (ie psychiatric illness is treated like any other personal injury) presumably because the privity of contract doctrine prevents the floodgates being opened.[110]

5.62 As the floodgates objection, in its most important sense, is not in play, we would expect the law to continue to develop by allowing claims by primary victims for psychiatric illness in a variety of situations (and irrespective of whether the illness

[106] The leading case is *Hedley Byrne & Co Ltd v Heller & Partners Ltd* [1964] AC 465.

[107] (1994) 144 NLJ 1659; see paras 2.49-2.50 above.

[108] See para 2.51 above.

[109] Ie other than those covered by propositions 3, 5 and 6 in para 2.3 above.

[110] See para 1.5 above.

is shock-induced or not). We see no valid reason to object to such a development. More specifically, we see no good reason why the *Walker* case should be regarded as incorrectly decided. On the contrary, the reasoning of Colman J seems to us to constitute a logical and just application of the law on safety at work to psychiatric illness.

5.63   We are therefore of the provisional view that, subject to standard defences,[111] there should be liability where an employer has negligently overburdened its employee with work thereby foreseeably causing him or her to suffer a psychiatric illness. Do consultees agree with this provisional view? If they do not agree, please would they give their reasons.

(7) Is legislation required in relation to negligently inflicted psychiatric illness?

5.64   There remains for determination the question whether reform of the law on psychiatric illness should be left to the courts or whether legislation is required. On the one hand, there may be a danger that legislative limits to recovery would be unduly rigid; and it can be argued that the common law on psychiatric illness can be expected to develop incrementally, as it has done in the past, so that any unwarranted restrictions that exist at present may in time be removed.

5.65   On the other hand, our provisional view, as we have explained above,[112] is that in respect of the central area of secondary victims - where the defendant has negligently injured or imperilled someone other than the plaintiff, and the plaintiff, as a result, has foreseeably suffered a psychiatric illness - the limits laid down or confirmed by the House of Lords in *Alcock* are too restrictive. After *Alcock* it is simply not open to courts below the House of Lords to decide, for example, that the test of perception through one's own unaided senses can be relaxed in respect of those with a close tie of love and affection to the primary victim.

5.66   The speeches in *Alcock* have also left the law uncertain. For example, they contained dicta suggesting that in certain circumstances damages might be recovered by bystanders and might be recovered by relatives who see a disaster on television.[113] But the necessary circumstances were left vague. Such uncertainty tends to promote litigation. As Michael Jones comments, some of the objections to *Alcock* "might be overcome if *Alcock* had succeeded in fixing a 'bright line' rule, which increased certainty in the law. Unfortunately it does not even achieve this ... Greater certainty could be achieved by adopting legislation similar to that of New South Wales."[114]

---

[111] See para 2.2 n 8 above.

[112] See paras 5.7-5.52 above.

[113] See paras 2.24 and 2.38 above.

[114] M Jones, *Textbook on Torts* (4th ed 1993) p 111.

5.67   Moreover, there is a strong case for arguing that the sort of issues in play in relation to questions of recovery by secondary victims - where "policy" restrictions on the "principle" of compensation for negligently caused harm are required - are particularly well-suited to legislative control. For example, we have considered it important in reaching our provisional views to know whether the medical literature and surveys support the central "policy" fear that the floodgates of litigation would be opened if one simply treated psychiatric illness like any other personal injury. This sort of information - and, particularly importantly, the views of a wide-ranging body of consultees that we are able to elicit through this paper - is not easily available, if at all, to the judiciary when they decide individual cases.

5.68   We also consider it relevant that both Lord Oliver and Lord Scarman have called for legislative intervention in relation to liability to secondary victims[115] and also that there has been legislation in this area in several Australian jurisdictions.[116]

5.69   **Our provisional view is that legislation is required to reform the law in the central area where the defendant has negligently injured or imperilled someone other than the plaintiff and the plaintiff, as a result, has foreseeably suffered a psychiatric illness. In contrast, we do not at present believe that it would be sensible to attempt to codify in a comprehensive legislative scheme the whole of the law on negligently inflicted psychiatric illness. We ask consultees whether they agree with those provisional views and generally whether they consider that any reforms they support should be implemented by legislation or should be left to incremental judicial development.**

5.70   If there were to be legislation governing liability in cases of psychiatric illness consequent on injury to, or fear for the safety of, another person, a further question would arise as to the relationship between that legislation and the common law in that area. It is to be noted, for example, that the Australian statutes have been interpreted as leaving untouched a plaintiff's right to bring a claim at common law.[117] This may be thought to have the advantage of avoiding a legislative freezing of the law. On the other hand, it may be argued that for any new legislation to be without prejudice to a plaintiff's rights at common law would render the law unnecessarily complex and uncertain and, in some circumstances, might encourage claimants needlessly to frame actions both under the statute and at common law. **We invite the views of consultees on this question.**

[115] See para 1.8 above.

[116] See Appendix, paras 15-21 below.

[117] See Appendix para 20.

PART VI
SUMMARY OF RECOMMENDATIONS AND CONSULTATION ISSUES

6.1 In this paper we have raised a large number of questions on this complex topic, and we have formed a provisional view on many of them. Our overall opinion, subject to the views of consultees, is that the central part of the law in relation to negligently inflicted psychiatric illness is in need of reform, and that the reform should be brought about by way of statute. We set out below a summary of our questions and provisional recommendations on which we invite the view of consultees.

(1) The abandonment of liability for negligently inflicted "pure" psychiatric illness

6.2 Do consultees agree with our provisional view that there should continue to be liability for negligently inflicted psychiatric illness that does not arise from a physical injury to the plaintiff? If they do not agree, please would they give their reasons. (paragraph 5.3)

(2) A requirement of actual or apprehended physical injury to the plaintiff

6.3 It was formerly a necessary condition of liability that the psychiatric illness sustained by the plaintiff should have arisen as a result of actual or apprehended physical injury to the plaintiff. Do consultees agree with our provisional view that that requirement should not be reintroduced? If they do not agree, please would they give their reasons. (paragraphs 5.4-5.6)

(3) The law where the defendant has negligently injured or imperilled someone other than the plaintiff, and the plaintiff, as a result, has foreseeably suffered a psychiatric illness

(i) Reasonable foreseeability as a sufficient test for the duty of care

6.4 Do consultees agree with our provisional conclusion that special limitations over and above reasonable foreseeability should continue to be applied to claims for psychiatric illness where the defendant has negligently injured or imperilled someone other than the plaintiff and the plaintiff, as a result, has suffered a psychiatric illness? If they do not agree, please would they give their reasons. (paragraphs 5.7-5.12)

(ii) The assumption, in applying the reasonable foreseeability test, that the plaintiff is a person of reasonable fortitude

6.5 We ask consultees: (a) whether they regard the emphasis on the plaintiff's reasonable fortitude as a restriction special to claims for psychiatric illness or, on the contrary, as no more than an application in the realm of psychiatric illness of the standard approach to reasonable foreseeability in personal injury cases; (b) whether the law should continue to assume that the plaintiff is a person of reasonable fortitude or, on the contrary, whether they consider it unsatisfactory to distinguish between reasonable fortitude and abnormal sensitivity. (paragraph 5.13)

(iii) The establishing of a close tie of love and affection between the plaintiff and the primary victim

6.6   We ask consultees whether there should be: (a) a fixed list of qualifying relationships of close love and affection; or (b) a list of relationships in which there is a rebuttable presumption of a close tie of love and affection, while also allowing a plaintiff not on that list to prove a close tie of love and affection; or (c) a list of relationships in which there is a rebuttable presumption of a close tie of love and affection, while not allowing a plaintiff outside that list to prove a close tie of love and affection; or (d) no list at all, so that a plaintiff has to prove on the facts of each case a close tie of love and affection; or (e) an approach different to any of (a) to (d) for establishing a close tie of love and affection between the plaintiff and the primary victim? (paragraphs 5.14-5.17)

6.7   We consider provisionally that if there is to be a list of relationships of close love and affection (whether fixed or rebuttable) it should include, at least, brothers and sisters, de facto spouses and those in a stable homosexual relationship in addition to spouses, children and parents (including anyone treated by the primary victim as a child of the family or as a parent). We ask consultees whether they agree with this provisional proposal; and whether they have any other suggestions to make as to the content of such a list. (paragraphs 5.18-5.19)

6.8   As regards the content of the proof of a close tie of love and affection, do consultees agree with our provisional view that it is sufficient to say that the plaintiff must prove a close tie of love and affection to the primary victim? If they do not agree, what do they suggest instead? (paragraph 5.20)

(iv) The abandonment of the requirements of closeness in time and space, and of perception through one's own unaided senses, where there is a close tie of love and affection between the plaintiff and the primary victim

6.9   Do consultees agree with our provisional central proposal that the requirements of closeness in time and space, and perception through one's own unaided senses, should be abandoned where there is a close tie of love and affection between the plaintiff and the primary victim? If consultees disagree with this provisional view we ask: (a) do they disagree because they fear that an abandonment of those two requirements would open the floodgates of litigation and, if so, do they have any evidence to support their fears?; and (b) would they propose any changes to the present requirements of closeness in time and space and perception through one's own unaided senses where there is a close tie of love and affection between the plaintiff and the primary victim? (Eg, should perception through live television qualify even if being told about the accident by a third party would not qualify?) (paragraphs 5.21-5.27)

6.10   The provisional proposal in the previous paragraph assumes that the reasonable foreseeability test must still be established. But we also ask consultees whether they support the different approach in Australian statutes of allowing plaintiffs within certain degrees of relationship to claim without having to establish that he or she is owed a duty of care. (paragraph 5.28)

(v) Plaintiffs without a close tie of love and affection to the primary victim

6.11   We invite the views of consultees as to whether mere bystanders should be able to recover damages for shock-induced psychiatric illness and, if so, in what circumstances. (paragraphs 5.29-5.30)

6.12   We ask consultees whether they agree with our provisional view that it would be unhelpful to lay down in legislation a definition of what counts as a rescue. We also invite the views of consultees as to whether professional rescuers should be precluded from recovering damages for negligently inflicted psychiatric illness sustained in the course of carrying out their duties; and, if not so precluded, we ask for views as to whether the same legal principles should be applied to determine the recovery of damages for negligently inflicted psychiatric illness by professional rescuers as are applied to ordinary rescuers. (paragraphs 5.31-5.35)

6.13   Do consultees agree with our provisional view that there should be a rule permitting recovery for psychiatric illness by involuntary participants for psychiatric illness as set out by Lord Oliver in *Alcock*?[1] If they do not agree, please would they give their reasons. (paragraphs 5.36-5.37)

(vi) The requirement (in secondary victim cases) that the psychiatric illness must have been shock-induced

6.14   We invite the views of consultees as to whether the requirement, in secondary victim cases, that the psychiatric illness must have been shock-induced, should be abandoned. (paragraphs 5.38-5.40)

(vii) A requirement that the psychiatric illness should be of a particular severity

6.15   Do consultees agree with our provisional view that damages for psychiatric illness should continue to be recoverable irrespective of whether the psychiatric illness is of a particular severity? If they do not agree, please would they give their reasons. (paragraphs 5.41-5.44)

(viii) The primary victim is the defendant

6.16   We ask consultees (a) should there be a bar to the recovery of damages for psychiatric illness where the primary victim is the defendant?; and, if so, (b) what should be the solution to the difficulty relating to contribution articulated by Lord Oliver in *Alcock*? (paragraphs 5.45-5.51)

---

[1]   [1992] 1 AC 310, 408.

(ix) The communication of true news as a possible break in the chain of causation between the negligence of the defendant and the plaintiff's psychiatric illness consequent on the communication of that news

6.17   Do consultees agree with our provisional view that normal principles of causation can satisfactorily resolve the question as to whether the communication of true news breaks the chain of causation between the negligence of the defendant, which caused the accident to the primary victim, and the plaintiff's psychiatric illness consequent on the communication of the news? If they do not agree, please would they give their reasons. (paragraph 5.52)

(4) The law where the defendant has negligently damaged or imperilled property belonging to the plaintiff or to a third party and the plaintiff, as a result, has foreseeably suffered a psychiatric illness

6.18   We ask consultees: (a) whether they agree with our provisional view that where psychiatric illness is consequent on damage, or danger, to the property of someone other than the plaintiff, criteria analogous to, but no less restrictive than, those applied where human safety or injury to another is involved, should be insisted on; (b) whether in that situation (ie where the psychiatric illness arises from damage to, or fear for, property belonging to someone other than the plaintiff) they would be in favour of retaining all three proximity requirements (ie relationship to the property, closeness in time and space, and perception through one's own unaided senses) and also the requirement that the psychiatric illness must have been shock-induced; (c) whether they consider that psychiatric illness consequent on damage, or danger, to one's own property should be equated with psychiatric illness consequent on personal injury, or danger, to oneself so that no special restrictions, over and above reasonable foreseeability, should be applied, and if not what they consider the special restrictions should be. (paragraphs 5.53-5.56)

(5) Liability for the negligent communication of news to the plaintiff foreseeably causing him or her to suffer a psychiatric illness

6.19   We ask consultees whether there should be liability for the negligent communication of news to the plaintiff causing him or her a foreseeable psychiatric illness. In particular we ask: (a) do consultees agree with our provisional view that the existence of a duty of care should not rest on foreseeability alone?; (b) if there are circumstances in which liability should be imposed, what are those circumstances?; (c) should a distinction be drawn depending on whether the news conveyed is true or false?; (d) should a further distinction be drawn between communication by the media to the public at large (although the information itself may specifically affect the plaintiff) and communication by officials and other individuals to specific individuals? (paragraphs 5.57-5.60)

(6) An employer's liability in the tort of negligence to its employee for a psychiatric illness foreseeably caused by overburdening the employee with work

6.20 Do consultees agree with our provisional view that, subject to standard defences, there should be liability where an employer has negligently overburdened its employee with work thereby foreseeably causing him or her to suffer a psychiatric illness? If they do not agree, please would they give their reasons. (paragraphs 5.61-5.63)

(7) The need for legislation in relation to negligently inflicted psychiatric illness

6.21 Do consultees agree with our provisional views: (a) that legislation is required to reform the law in the central area where the defendant has negligently injured or imperilled someone other than the plaintiff and the plaintiff, as a result, has suffered a foreseeable psychiatric illness?; (b) that it would not be sensible to attempt to codify in a comprehensive legislative scheme the whole of the law on negligently inflicted psychiatric illness? We also ask consultees generally whether they consider that any reforms they support should be implemented by legislation or should be left to incremental judicial development. (paragraphs 5.64-5.69)

6.22 We invite the views of consultees as to whether any legislation that they favour should be without prejudice to a plaintiff's rights at common law. (paragraph 5.70)

Questions from Parts I-IV

6.23 We would welcome the views of consultees as to the torts (or, conceivably, non-tortious causes of action) in respect of which liability for psychiatric illness attracts special restrictions (ie restrictions that are not applied to liability for physical injury). In particular we would be pleased to hear from practitioners who have encountered such special restrictions in respect of claims for psychiatric illness not based on the tort of negligence. We would also be grateful for views as to whether we are correct in our understanding that, in actions for breach of contract, no special restrictions are placed on the recovery of damages for psychiatric illness and whether, if that is so, consultees consider, as we do, that that is a justified approach for the law to take. (paragraphs 1.5-1.6)

6.24 We ask consultees: are the problems of assessing damages for psychiatric illness thought to be so much greater than for other types of personal injury that a different method or regime should be adopted for the assessment of damages for psychiatric illness than is adopted for assessing damages for other types of personal injury? (paragraph 2.55)

6.25 We invite general comments on the summary of medical research in Part III of this paper. More specifically we invite the views of those with expertise in the field: (a) as to whether they consider that our summary of the relevant medical background and research, and our conclusions, are fair and accurate and, if not, why not; (b) as to what they believe to be the incidence of psychiatric illnesses caused by injury to, or fear for the safety of, others and as to whether a survey could sensibly be carried out on that specific issue; and (c) as to any other medical considerations they believe we should be taking into account. (paragraph 3.16)

General

6.26   We invite consultees to comment on any other aspect of liability for psychiatric illness which they consider relevant to the general purpose of this paper, but on which we have not specifically sought the views of consultees.

APPENDIX
OTHER JURISDICTIONS[1]

SCOTLAND

1. The law relating to negligently inflicted psychiatric illness bears similarities to that in England[2] despite the different theoretical foundations of the two jurisdictions. Thus, the pursuer must establish that he or she is suffering from mental injury caused by shock, going beyond a mere emotional reaction.[3] However, in common with other jurisdictions that are also heavily influenced by Roman law, the Scottish courts have exhibited a greater reluctance to roll back the boundaries of recovery. For example, the requirement that the plaintiff must have been within the zone of physical danger was only abandoned in 1962.[4] The recent decision in *Robertson v Forth Road Bridge Joint Board (No 2)*,[5] discussed below, indicates that the Scottish courts will interpret the House of Lords' decision in *Alcock* quite narrowly.

2. The category of claimants who have succeeded in recovering damages have included parents,[6] children[7] and adult siblings[8] of persons injured or killed as a result of the defendant's negligence. However, in *Robertson v Forth Road Bridge Joint Board (No 2)*[9] the Outer House interpreted the requirement of a close tie of love and affection laid down in *Alcock* as requiring "the closest ties of friendship or family".[10] In that

---

[1] This brief survey of the attitudes of some other jurisdictions to negligently inflicted psychiatric illness is by no means exhaustive, and we are aware that the questions discussed are also problematic in jurisdictions which we have not specifically discussed: see, eg, T Plewman's review, from a South African perspective, of N J Mullany and P R Handford, *op cit* (1994) 111 SALJ 213.

[2] *Bourhill v Young* [1943] AC 92, the first decision of the House of Lords to establish the principle of liability in the tort of negligence for shock-induced psychiatric illness, was an appeal from the Court of Session, although the plaintiff failed, on the facts of the case, to recover damages. *McLoughlin v O'Brian* is cited in *Gloag and Henderson* in support of the view that whether there is liability for psychiatric illness is essentially a question of reasonable foreseeability: A B Wilkinson and W A Wilson (eds), *Gloag and Henderson's Introduction to the Law of Scotland* (9th ed 1987) p 548. See also D M Walker, *The Law of Delict in Scotland* (2nd ed 1981) pp 679-680.

[3] *Wallace v Kennedy* 1908 16 SLT 485; *Simpson v Imperial Chemical Industries Ltd* 1983 SLT 601; *Harvey v Cairns* 1988 SCLR 254; 1989 SLT 107. See also *Moffatt v Secretary of State for Scotland* (1994, unreported).

[4] *McLinden v Richardson* 1962 SLT (Notes) 104. See N J Mullany and P R Handford, *Tort Liability for Psychiatric Damage* (1993) p 9.

[5] 1994 SLT 568 (OH).

[6] See eg *Morton v Wiseman* 1989 SCLR 365; *Lowrie v Carrington & Dewhurst Ltd* 1974 SLT (Notes) 11.

[7] Eg, *Jarvie v Sharp* 1992 SLT 350; *Greenwood v Muir* 1977 SLT (Notes) 71.

[8] Eg, *Clarke v McFadyen* 1989 Green's Weekly Digest 18-768; 1989 SCLR 792.

[9] 1994 SLT 568.

[10] *Ibid*, 572.

case, the pursuers were both working colleagues of the deceased. The first pursuer had been a colleague for most of his working life, and he also socialised with the deceased on a weekly basis; the second pursuer had been a colleague for some years. The deceased was blown by a strong gust of wind from the back of an open pick-up truck travelling over the Forth road bridge, fell over the side of the bridge and was killed. The truck was being driven by the first pursuer and followed in another vehicle by the second pursuer. It was held that neither had the necessary close tie of love and affection to the deceased.

3. The pursuers in *Robertson* also failed in their claims that they fell within the category of "involuntary participants" or that the accident was so horrific that they should succeed as "bystanders". The court held that the mere fact that they and the deceased were co-workers engaged in the same operation did not of itself warrant that they should be treated as participants in the accident, as the plaintiff was in the case of *Dooley v Cammell Laird & Co.*[11] In rejecting the pursuers' claims in the alternative capacity of "bystanders", the court relied on the recent Court of Appeal decision in *McFarlane v EE Caledonia Ltd*[12] in which the plaintiff failed on this basis even though the circumstances were "considerably more appalling".[13]

4. It appears that a plaintiff will not be successful in claiming damages where the primary victim is the defendant. In dicta in the Outer House in *Bourhill v Young*,[14] Lord Robertson ruled out liability for nervous shock caused to others in the hypothetical example of a window-cleaner falling and impaling himself on spiked railings due to his own negligence. In the previous case of *A v B's Trustees*,[15] the plaintiffs had recovered damages from the estate of their lodger after the lodger committed suicide in his lodgings, causing the plaintiffs to suffer psychiatric illness. This case has, however, been explained as being founded on contract, or alternatively on the fact that the lodger also caused some material damage to the premises.[16]

---

[11] [1951] 1 Lloyd's Rep 271. See para 2.28 above.

[12] [1994] 2 All ER 1. See para 2.24 above.

[13] 1994 SLT 568, 573. See J Blaikie, "Nervous Shock: Traumatised Fellow Workers and Bystanders" 1994 SLT (News) 297.

[14] 1941 SC 395, 399; affirmed by the House of Lords [1943] AC 92.

[15] 1906 13 SLT 830.

[16] *Bourhill v Young* [1943] AC 92, 120, *per* Lord Porter.

IRELAND

5.   The courts in Ireland were quicker than those in England to recognise liability for negligently inflicted psychiatric illness, with the two cases establishing that liability being decided in the nineteenth century.[17]

6.   Two recent cases have examined the issue of proximity where a close relation hears of the accident and finds her or his loved one badly injured in hospital. In *Mullally v Bus Eireann*[18] the plaintiff discovered that her husband and three sons had been injured in a bus crash which had killed three people and left many more injured. Shock set in when she was told the news. She travelled to the hospitals where they were being treated, where, several hours later, she found her husband and sons in a distressing condition. Conditions in the first of the hospitals were especially harrowing because of the number of victims of the accident being treated. One of the sons died some months later. It was held that the plaintiff was entitled to recover damages. Whilst believing that the proximity between the plaintiff and the accident brought her within the circumstances envisaged by Lord Wilberforce's speech in *McLoughlin*,[19] Denham J expressed preference for the approach of Lord Bridge in that case,[20] and she appeared to base her decision on the pure foreseeability of the psychiatric illness in the case rather than on any considerations of proximity.[21] *Mullally v Bus Eireann* was followed in *Kelly v Hennessy*[22] where the plaintiff had suffered psychiatric illness in similar circumstances. Again the shock began when the news of the accident was communicated to the plaintiff, and was followed by an extremely traumatic visit to the primary victim[23] in hospital. The plaintiff recovered damages. One of the cases cited in argument was *Alcock*, but there was no discussion of it in the judgment of Lavan J. It therefore seems likely that the "aftermath" doctrine has been extended in Irish law beyond its current limit in England.

AUSTRALIA
(1) Common law

7.   The concept of common law liability for negligently inflicted pure psychiatric illness was accepted by the High Court in *Bunyan v Jordan*,[24] in which Dixon J said that

---

[17]   *Bell v Great Northern Rly Co of Ireland* (1890) 26 LR Ir 428; *Byrne v Great Southern & Western Rly Co of Ireland* (1884) unreported (CA).

[18]   [1992] ILRM 722.

[19]   [1983] 1 AC 410, 422.

[20]   *Ibid*, 441-443.

[21]   [1992] ILRM 722, 731.

[22]   [1993] ILRM 530.

[23]   The plaintiff's husband.

[24]   (1937) 57 CLR 1.

he had "no doubt that [psychiatric] illness without more is a form of harm or damage sufficient for the purpose of any action on the case in which damage is the gist of the action, that is, supposing that the other ingredients of the cause of action are present,"[25] although the plaintiff failed on the facts. Shortly afterwards, the development of liability was checked in *Chester v Waverley Corporation*,[26] but subject to a strong dissenting judgment from Evatt J. Some thirty years later the trend towards wider liability was resumed in *Mount Isa Mines Ltd v Pusey*,[27] and the leading case is now *Jaensch v Coffey*.[28]

8. The facts in *Jaensch* were similar to *McLoughlin*. The plaintiff's husband was involved in an accident. He was taken to hospital and underwent repeated surgical treatment on the day of the injury. It was then doubtful whether he would survive, and this remained in doubt for several weeks. The plaintiff was not with her husband at the time of the injury, but she visited the hospital on the same day and was there for a long period on the following day. As a result partly of what she saw and partly of what she was told by hospital personnel she developed a severe psychiatric disorder. The plaintiff was successful in recovering damages, the High Court of Australia holding that the aftermath of the accident extended to the scene at the hospital during the period of immediate post-accident treatment. Gibbs CJ and Deane J went even further in intimating that a plaintiff might recover as a result of being *told* about the death or accident.[29] Brennan and Dawson JJ, on the other hand, thought that there was no liability for psychiatric illness brought about by mere communication by a third party.[30]

9. There is no rule that, when the plaintiff visits the primary victim in hospital, the victim must be witnessed by the plaintiff in much the same condition as at the scene

---

[25] *Ibid*, 16.

[26] (1939) 62 CLR 1. The plaintiff, a mother who had seen the body of her seven-year-old son being removed from a water-filled ditch, was held to be unable to recover damages for the resulting psychiatric illness on the ground of lack of foreseeability.

[27] (1970) 125 CLR 383.

[28] (1984) 155 CLR 549.

[29] (1984) 155 CLR 549, 555, 608. See also *Bassanese v Martin* (1982) 31 SASR 461; *Petrie v Dowling* [1989] Aust Torts Reports 68,811 - but see D Mendelson, "The Defendants' Liability for Negligently Caused Nervous Shock in Australia - Quo Vadis?" [1992] 18 Mon LR 16, 43, for an alternative explanation of *Petrie* as being within the "immediate aftermath" exception as defined in *Jaensch*. On liability *against the conveyer of news* for the negligent communication of *false* information, see *Barnes v Commonwealth of Australia* (1937) 37 SR (NSW) 511 (NSW Sup Ct), in which the plaintiff recovered damages from the government after she received a letter from a government office containing the incorrect statement that her husband had been admitted to a mental hospital, causing the plaintiff to suffer psychiatric illness. See also *Brown v Mount Barker Soldiers' Hospital Inc* [1934] SASR 128 (SA Sup Ct): see para 2.46 n 143 above.

[30] (1984) 155 CLR 549, 567, 612.

of the accident.[31] It also appears to be settled that, where the plaintiff sustains physical injury and is rendered unconscious in an accident in which a third party is seriously injured or killed, the plaintiff can recover damages for psychiatric illness sustained on merely being informed of that death or serious injury.[32]

10. The limitations on liability set by the proximity tests, and the effect of *Jaensch* on those limitations, are illustrated by the decision of the Supreme Court of Queensland in *Spence v Percy*.[33] In that case the plaintiff's twenty-year-old daughter was rendered permanently comatose by an accident caused by the defendant's negligence. The plaintiff was not present at the scene. She suffered anxiety and stress as a result of being told about the accident, and on visiting her daughter in hospital, and subsequently in the course of looking after her, during which there were a number of crises. However, she did not actually suffer psychiatric illness until after her daughter died, some three years later. Although the plaintiff succeeded at first instance, the defendant's appeal was allowed. It was held that the lapse of time between the accident and the onset of psychiatric illness meant that the illness occurred outside the aftermath of the accident, and the requirement of "causal proximity"[34] was not met.

11. The High Court in *Jaensch* did not resolve the question whether a plaintiff must have a close tie of love and affection to the primary victim, or be a rescuer[35] or involuntary participant,[36] in order to be able to recover. There was no doubt, of

---

[31] See, eg, *Petrie v Dowling* [1989] Aust Torts Reports 68,811 (plaintiff did not see the immediate post-accident state of her child's body); *Orman v Harrington* (unreported, SA Sup Ct, 30 April 1990, No 296 of 1990) (plaintiff did not visit victim until next day). See also Mullany and Handford, *op cit*, p 149. Cf the position in England (see paras 2.29-2.31 above.)

[32] See, eg, *Andrews v Williams* [1967] VR 831; *Regan v Harper* [1971] Qd R 191; *Gannon v Gray* [1973] Qd R 411; *Kohn v State Government Insurance Commission* (1976) 15 SASR 255; *Tsanaktsidis v Oulianoff* (1980) 24 SASR 500 (SA Sup Ct); *Jaensch v Coffey* (1984) 155 CLR 549, 609, *per* Deane J. Cf *Schneider v Eisovitch* [1960] 2 QB 430 (see para 2.34 above).

[33] [1992] 2 Qd R 299. See J Meredith, "Step by Cautious Step - A Recent Finding on Nervous Shock" [1991] Qld Law Soc J 427. See also the review of Mullany and Handford, *op cit* by B A Hocking (1994) Psychiatry Psychology and Law 59.

[34] *Jaensch v Coffey* (1984) 155 CLR 549, 606-607, *per* Deane J.

[35] *Mount Isa Mines Ltd v Pusey* (1970) 125 CLR 383. On the facts of that case the plaintiff was a rescuer albeit that the judgments tended to emphasise that he was a fellow employee. In *Jaensch v Coffey* (1984) 155 CLR 549, 561, 569, Brennan J emphasised that in *Pusey* the plaintiff was a rescuer.

[36] Whilst involuntary participation in an accident will most likely establish of itself a sufficiently proximate relationship between the parties, it seems that in Australia, as in England, the mere fact that the defendant is the employer of the plaintiff, or that the plaintiff and third party victim were co-workers, will not suffice to demonstrate the required proximity: *Wilks v Haines* [1991] Aust Torts Reports 68,649. See also Appendix, para 3 above. However, it was decided in *Miller v Royal Derwent Hospital Board of Management* [1992] Aust Torts Reports 61,483 (Tas Sup Ct) that where it is reasonably foreseeable that the event in question might be witnessed by a person standing in a special

course, that on the facts of that case, the plaintiff would have been eligible whatever the rule. Whilst one member of the High Court[37] was inclined to think that the relationship between the plaintiff and the primary victim was of great importance, two of the judges would not have ruled out recovery by a mere bystander unrelated to the primary victim if the circumstances were unusual or exceptional.[38] It is probably correct to say that, although it will not be decisive, proximity of relationship will be relevant in applying the test of foreseeability.[39] However, there does not appear to have been an Australian decision as yet permitting recovery of damages by ordinary bystanders who perceive a traumatic event or accident.[40]

12. As regards those with a tie of love and affection to the primary victim, recovery has for the most part been limited in practice in Australia to persons within the immediate family nucleus. However, there are a few isolated examples in some jurisdictions of recovery in respect of persons who were not within this relationship. In *Storm v Geeves*,[41] Burbury CJ in the Tasmanian Supreme Court extended recovery to include siblings,[42] and in *Kohn v State Government Insurance Commission*[43] the plaintiff recovered damages for psychiatric illness and distress consequent on being informed of the death of a close friend as a result of injuries sustained in the same accident.[44] Where the plaintiff's psychiatric illness is attributable to concern about the death, injury or peril of the defendant himself or herself, damages will not be recoverable.[45]

13. Despite the relaxation of the law in some respects, it is still true to say that the plaintiff must establish that he or she is suffering from a recognised psychiatric

relationship to the victim, the duty of care is to be defined by reference to any heightened susceptibility to injury expected to be produced by the fact of that special relationship (the plaintiff in *Miller* was a nurse at the hospital in which the victim was a patient).

[37] (1984) 155 CLR 549, 555-556, *per* Gibbs CJ.

[38] (1984) 155 CLR, 549, 605-606, *per* Deane J; 570, *per* Brennan J. See also *Mount Isa Mines Ltd v Pusey* (1970) 125 CLR 383, 404, *per* Windeyer J; 416-417, *per* Walsh J.

[39] *Jaensch v Coffey* (1984) 155 CLR 549, 605-606, *per* Deane J.

[40] See, however, the settlement cited by Mullany and Handford, *op cit*, p 130, n 119. See generally F Trindade and P Cane, *The Law of Torts in Australia* (2nd ed 1993) pp 344-345.

[41] [1965] Tas SR 252.

[42] *Ibid*, 266-267.

[43] (1976) 15 SASR 255 (SA Sup Ct).

[44] However, the plaintiff also sustained serious physical injury in the accident so that the court's approach might be justified on the basis that the plaintiff also suffered physical injury.

[45] *Jaensch v Coffey* (1984) 155 CLR 549, 604, *per* Deane J; *Harrison v State Government Insurance Office* [1985] Aust Torts Reports para 80-723 (Queensland Supreme Ct); *Klug v Motor Accidents Insurance Board* [1991] Aust Torts Reports para 81-1345 (Tasmania Supreme Ct). See Mullany and Handford, *op cit*, pp 215-220.

illness attributable to shock caused by the defendant's negligence to be able to recover for psychiatric illness in Australia at common law.[46] However, the Australian courts now appear to be beginning to recognise the possibility that an employer may be liable for psychiatric illness resulting from work-related stress, even though the stress inducing that illness is continuous rather than a single shock.[47] But where, in an employment context, psychiatric illness follows a single traumatic event, it will still have to be proved, as in *Jaensch* and similar cases, that the psychiatric illness is caused by sudden shock brought on by perception of the event and not, for example, by a more gradual anxiety in relation to the event's consequences.[48]

14.   As regards the assessment of damages for psychiatric illness, the separation test (exemplified in England by *Hinz v Berry*)[49] has been under some attack. In *Richters v Motor Tyre Service Pty Ltd*,[50] the Queensland Supreme Court held that because it was the shock of witnessing the events in question (and not grief alone) which "tipped the balance" and drove the plaintiff to her psychiatric state, the "whole degree" of her mental condition was compensatable; and in *Harrison v State Government Insurance Office*,[51] the Queensland Supreme Court dismissed the test as a "meaningless and unrealistic exercise". In *De Franceshi v Storrier*,[52] the Supreme Court of the Australian Capital Territory described as an "artificial exercise" the process of separating out those elements in the plaintiff's condition which related

---

[46]   *Jaensch v Coffey* (1984) 155 CLR 549, 566-567, *per* Brennan J, 587-588, *per* Deane J; *Mount Isa Mines Ltd v Pusey* (1970) 125 CLR 383, 394, *per* Windeyer J; *Pavlovic v Commonwealth Bank of Australia* (1991) 56 SASR 587 (SA Sup Ct). See also *Andrewartha v Andrewartha (No 1)* (1987) 44 SASR 1; *Anderson v Smith* (1990) 101 FLR 34; *Pratt and Goldsmith v Pratt* [1975] VR 378; *Swan v Williams (Demolition) Pty Limited* (1989) 9 NSWLR 172.

[47]   *Gillespie v Commonwealth of Australia* (1991) 104 ACTR 1 (Australian Capital Territory Supreme Court), in which the plaintiff, an employee of the Department of Foreign Affairs, suffered a breakdown following an extremely stressful posting to the diplomatic mission in Caracas. However, recovery was denied to the plaintiff on the basis that the defendant had complied with its duty of care. See also *Wodrow v Commonwealth of Australia* (1993) 45 FCR 52 (Federal Ct), in which the plaintiff again failed on the facts (Cf paras 2.49-2.50 above). Note also the interesting case of *Campbelltown City Council v Mackay* (1989) 15 NSWLR 501 in which damages were awarded for gradually sustained psychiatric illness consequent on damage to the plaintiff's property (see para 2.44 n 138 above).

[48]   See *Sandstrom v Commonwealth of Australia* (1994; Federal Court) and *Dinnison v Commonwealth of Australia* (1994; Federal Court). See also *Dingwall v Commonwealth of Australia* (1994; Federal Court) in which Foster J declined to consider this question. All three cases arose out of psychiatric illness alleged to have been suffered by former servicemen as a result of their presence at the nuclear test explosions at Maralinga, South Australia in 1956 and 1957.

[49]   [1970] 2 QB 40 (see para 2.8 above).

[50]   [1972] Qd R 9.

[51]   [1985] Aust Torts Reports para 80-723 (Vasta J).

[52]   (1988) 85 ACTR 1. This action was brought under s 24(1) of the Law Reform (Miscellaneous Provisions) Ordinance 1955 (see para 16 below), although the statutory nature of the claim did not affect the quantum of damages.

to the psychiatric illness and those which sprang merely from natural concern, but it nevertheless accepted that the exercise had to be undertaken.[53] Similarly, Deane J in *Jaensch v Coffey* thought that, where psychiatric illness resulted from what was seen or heard at the scene of the accident or its aftermath, the fact that the injury was subsequently aggravated as a result of the plaintiff being told of the deterioration or death of the person injured should neither preclude recovery nor require apportionment between causes.[54]

(2) Statutory modification

15. Legislative provisions in New South Wales, Victoria, South Australia, the Australian Capital Territory and the Northern Territory provide that a person will not be precluded from recovering damages merely because the injury complained of arose wholly or in part from psychiatric illness.[55] These provisions were enacted in response to such restrictive decisions as *Victorian Railways Commissioners v Coultas*[56] and *Chester v Waverley Corporation*[57] which virtually excluded negligently inflicted psychiatric illness as a head of damage. However, the common law has since caught up, with the effect that the absence of similar legislative provisions in other states is of no practical importance.

16. The legislation in New South Wales, the Australian Capital Territory and the Northern Territory, however, went beyond merely removing any bar on claims for psychiatric illness. It also laid down some relatively liberal rights of recovery for wrongfully inflicted mental or nervous shock[58] (although there are now different statutory rules in relation to motor accidents and workplace accidents in New South Wales).[59] This legislation provides that the liability of a person in respect of injury caused by an act, neglect or default by which another person is killed, injured or put in peril extends to include liability for injury arising wholly or in part from mental or nervous shock sustained by a parent or the spouse (or in New South Wales and the Northern Territory, the de facto spouse)[60] of the person killed, injured or put

---

[53]   *Ibid*, 8, *per* Miles CJ.

[54]   (1984) 155 CLR 549, 609.

[55]   **NSW** Law Reform (Miscellaneous Provisions) Act 1944, s 3; **Victoria** Wrongs Act 1958, s 23; **South Australia** Wrongs Act 1936, s 28; **Northern Territory** Law Reform (Miscellaneous Provisions) Act 1956, s 24; **Australian Capital Territory** Law Reform (Miscellaneous Provisions) Ordinance 1955, s 23.

[56]   (1888) 13 App Cas 222.

[57]   (1939) 62 CLR 1.

[58]   **NSW** Law Reform (Miscellaneous Provisions) Act 1944, s 4; **Northern Territory** Law Reform (Miscellaneous Provisions) Act 1956, s 25; **Australian Capital Territory** Law Reform (Miscellaneous Provisions) Ordinance 1955, s 24.

[59]   See para 21 below.

[60]   **NSW** Law Reform (Miscellaneous Provisions) Act 1944, s 4(5); **Northern Territory** Law Reform (Miscellaneous Provisions) Act 1956, s 25(1).

in peril; or by any other member of the family within whose sight or hearing the person was killed, injured or put in peril. "Member of the family" is defined to include child, brother, sister, half-brother or half-sister of the person killed, injured or put in peril. "Parent" includes father, mother, grandfather, grandmother, stepfather, stepmother and any person standing *in loco parentis* to another. "Child" includes son, daughter, grandson, granddaughter, stepson, stepdaughter and any person to whom another stands *in loco parentis*.[61]

17. The main effect of that legislation is a liberalising one, removing as it does from the plaintiff, in specified cases, the burden of proving, as is necessary under the Australian common law, that the defendant ought reasonably to have foreseen the possibility of causing the plaintiff injury through shock.[62] In other words, the legislation dispenses with the need for the claimant to establish an independent duty. Under these provisions the parent, husband or wife of the person killed, injured or put in peril may now recover regardless of how he or she acquired knowledge of the accident, and regardless of any spatial or temporal proximity to the accident. It is sufficient, for example, to be told of the accident by a third party. Even in respect of other members of the family, the burden of proof is made substantially lighter than it would be at common law, in so far as the plaintiff may recover without having to establish the quality of the relationship with the primary victim. It is worth noting the lack of reported cases in which the liability of the defendant to the plaintiff under the statute has been disputed, where the plaintiff has suffered psychiatric illness and the defendant's negligence has been established. In the New South Wales case of *Smee v Tibbetts*,[63] for example, the mother of the primary victim suffered psychiatric illness after she was informed by the police of her daughter's death in a road accident. The appeal turned on the question whether the defendant was liable to the mother's husband[64] for loss of consortium. The liability of the defendant to the *mother* was not disputed, even though similar facts would not, then or now, enable recovery at common law in England or in many other jurisdictions.

---

[61] **NSW** Law Reform (Miscellaneous Provisions) Act 1944, s 4(5); **Northern Territory** Law Reform (Miscellaneous Provisions) Act 1956, s 23; **Australian Capital Territory** Law Reform (Miscellaneous Provisions) Ordinance 1955, s 22.

[62] P Heffey, "The Negligent Infliction of Nervous Shock in Road and Industrial Accidents: Part II" (1974) 48 ALJ 240, 248.

[63] (1953) 53 SR (NSW) 391.

[64] The primary victim's father, who was informed of the death at the same time, but was unable to establish that he had himself suffered a psychiatric illness.

18.   The common law notion of actionable psychiatric illness is retained in so far as the plaintiff's illness must amount to a medically recognised one[65] attributable to shock. The plaintiff must also establish causation under the legislation. The test of causation will presumably be sufficient to exclude liability where there is intervention by a malicious or negligent third party, in the reporting of an accident, for example. The defendant must also have been in breach of duty to the person killed, injured or put in peril,[66] although, as at common law, liability to the immediate victim is not a condition for recovery by the plaintiff.[67] The plaintiff's right of action arising out of the statute is an independent one, not merely a right to sue derived from the primary victim's right of action.[68]

19.   The legislation anticipates the existence of a three-party situation. The plaintiff is therefore precluded from recovering under the legislation where psychiatric illness results from fear for his or her *own* safety, or where this is attributable to anticipated or actual harm inflicted by the defendant upon him or herself.[69] The third party must also be placed in actual danger and a mere belief that she or he is in danger will not suffice, no matter how reasonable the belief, although it is not necessary for the primary victim to have sustained actual injury. The legislation also does not extend to allowing recovery for psychiatric illness resulting from fear of harm to persons unrelated to the person killed, injured or imperilled, or to non-human interests.

20.   The question inevitably arose for decision whether the legislation excluded all other causes of action for negligently inflicted psychiatric illness or whether it merely created a supplementary cause of action so that those who could not bring their claims within the statutory provisions could bring a claim at common law. In

---

[65] See NSW Parliamentary Debates, 1944, vol 175, Mr McKell, p 521. See also P Heffey, "The Negligent Infliction of Nervous Shock in Road and Industrial Accidents: Part II" (1974) 48 ALJ 240, 249, n 39.

[66] *Scala v Mammolitti* (1965) 114 CLR 153: the plaintiff must show that the defendant's act, neglect or default was "in some sense wrongful" (162, *per* Windeyer J) or "wrongful in the sense that it was in breach of a duty owed to the person 'killed, injured or put in peril'" (161, *per* Menzies J; 157, *per* Kitto J) or "careless" (158, *per* Taylor J). See also *Anderson v Liddy* (1949) 49 SR (NSW) 320, 323. Heffey, however, submits that there will be cases where the plaintiff should be able to recover where the defendant's act etc is not wrongful in respect of the accident victim: "The Negligent Infliction of Nervous Shock in Road and Industrial Accidents: Part II" (1974) 48 ALJ 240, 253.

[67] In *Scala v Mammolitti* (1965) 114 CLR 153, the High Court of Australia decided that the reference to "liability" in s 4(1) of the NSW Law Reform (Miscellaneous Provisions) Act 1944 referred not to an existing liability but to amenability to claims. Nor was the court of the opinion that a prior judgment against the accident victim barred the plaintiff from bringing an action under the statute for psychiatric illness resulting from the same incident.

[68] *Smee v Tibbetts* (1953) 53 SR (NSW) 391; *State Rail Authority of New South Wales v Sharp* [1981] 1 NSWLR 240.

[69] See, eg, *Ball v Winslett* (1958) SR (NSW) 149.

Stergiou v Stergiou [70] the Supreme Court of the Australian Capital Territory held that the legislation in that territory did not exclusively govern liability for psychiatric illness, and the prevailing opinion is that the legislation should be understood as being supplementary to, rather than a substitute for, the common law. [71] Therefore, it is open to non-relatives, for example, and to relatives who do not see or hear the accident itself but rather witness its aftermath, to bring a claim at common law for psychiatric illness.

21. In New South Wales and South Australia there is legislation, applying to certain motor vehicle accidents, which (at least in New South Wales) [72] restricts the circumstances in which a plaintiff can recover for psychiatric illness. [73] In New South Wales, no damages for "psychological or psychiatric injury" are to be awarded in respect of a motor accident except in favour of two categories of person: first, those who suffered injury in the accident; and, secondly, parents, spouse (including a "de facto partner"), [74] brothers, sisters or children of the person injured. [75] In South Australia no damages for "mental or nervous shock" are to be awarded in respect of a motor accident except in favour of persons physically injured in the accident or the parent, spouse or child of a person killed, injured or endangered in the

[70]   [1987] Aust Torts Reports 68,435 (Gallop J).

[71]   In *Stergiou* the plaintiff was a passenger in a car which collided with a cyclist. The plaintiff sought damages for her alleged psychiatric illness consequent on the perception that the cyclist may have been killed. Gallop J held that although the plaintiff could not bring herself within the relevant statutory provision, she was entitled to maintain an action on the basis of the common law. In the end, the action failed because no demonstrable psychiatric illness had been proved. See also *Scala v Mammolitti* (1965) 114 CLR 153, 157, *per* Kitto J (High Ct of Australia, on appeal from NSW Supreme Ct) and *Wilks v Haines* [1991] Aust Torts Reports 68, 649 (NSW Supreme Ct).

[72]   As South Australia did not enact liberalising provisions generally, the new provisions are in some respects less restrictive than the previous (common) law.

[73]   In New South Wales the purpose behind the Motor Accidents Act 1988 was to bring back the common law in respect of personal injuries suffered in motor accidents, which had been replaced in the Transport Accidents Compensation Act 1987 by the "TransCover" compensation system: see *Motor Accidents: the Act and Background Papers* (NSW Attorney-General's Department, 1989). We have been unable to find any specific reason for s 77 of the Motor Accidents Act 1988 and it appears that the section received no mention in Parliamentary debates. We are grateful to the New South Wales Law Reform Commission for their help on this issue.

[74]   "De facto partner" is defined, in relation to a woman, as a man who is living with the woman as her husband on a bona fide domestic basis although not married to her, or, if the woman's death is caused by the fault of the owner or driver of a motor vehicle in the use or operation of the vehicle, a man who, immediately before the date of the woman's death, was living with the woman on such a basis. It is defined similarly, mutatis mutandis, in relation to a man: **NSW** Motor Accidents Act 1988, s 3(1).

[75]   **NSW** Motor Accidents Act 1988, s 77. This interpretation of s 77 is supported by Mullany and Handford, *op cit*, p 244. But the wording of the section is tortuous: a possible alternative interpretation taken, for example, by J Fleming, *The Law of Torts* (8th ed 1992) p 164, is that anyone, even if not a friend or relative, present at the scene of the accident can recover for psychiatric injury.

accident.[76] In New South Wales there are also statutory provisions limiting recovery for psychological or psychiatric injuries resulting from accidents suffered in the course of employment.[77]

NEW ZEALAND[78]

22.   In recent years very little personal injury litigation has taken place in New Zealand owing to the fact that a statutory accident compensation scheme was introduced there in 1974, under the Accident Compensation Act 1972, as amended by the Accident Compensation Amendment Act 1973. The scheme and interim amendments were re-enacted in the Accident Compensation Act 1982. Where cover is provided by the scheme the common law right to claim damages is statutorily barred.

23.   The statutory scheme focuses on "personal injury by accident". This term, which was not defined by the Accident Compensation Act 1982, was construed very widely and the boundaries of the scheme were greatly extended to include, for example, psychiatric illness unaccompanied by physical injury.[79] However, significant changes to the scheme came into effect on 1 July 1992 under the Accident Rehabilitation and Compensation Insurance Act 1992 ("ARCIA 1992"), which sought to curb the costs of the statutory scheme which were seen to be escalating.

24.   ARCIA 1992 applies to personal injuries occurring in New Zealand on or after 1 July 1992. The limits of recovery under the statutory scheme have been severely circumscribed by this Act. The ARCIA 1992 bars recovery for mental injury unless it is accompanied by physical injury. "Personal injury" and "accident" are separately defined. "Personal injury" is defined as (i) the death of, or physical injuries to, a person, and any mental injury suffered by that person which is an outcome of those physical injuries to that person; and (ii) any mental or nervous shock suffered by a person which is an outcome of certain sexual offences listed in Schedule 1 to the Act.[80] "Mental injury" is defined as a clinically significant behavioural, psychological

---

[76]   **South Australia** Wrongs Act 1936, s 35a(1)(c), which was brought into force in 1986. In *Compensation for Victims of Motor Vehicle Accidents* (Report No 52, 1987) p 45 the Law Reform Commission of Tasmania recommended the adoption of a provision similar to s 35a(1)(c) of the South Australia Wrongs Act 1936.

[77]   **NSW** Workers Compensation Act 1987, s 151P (amended by Workers Compensation (Benefits) Amendment Act 1989).

[78]   See generally, R Tobin, "Nervous Shock: The Common Law; Accident Compensation?" [1992] NZLJ 282. We are grateful to the New Zealand Law Commission for its assistance in compiling this section.

[79]   *Accident Compensation Commission v E* [1992] 2 NZLR 426.

[80]   ARCIA 1992, ss 4 and 8(3).

or cognitive dysfunction.[81] Before ARCIA 1992, "accident" bore its common law meaning, namely, an unlooked for mishap or an untoward event which is not expected or designed, but in ARCIA 1992 the word is defined as meaning a specific event or series of events that involves the application of a force or resistance external to the human body but not including any gradual process.[82]

25.   Subject to a limited exception which covers the victims of sexual assaults, therefore, "nervous shock" will only be covered by the new statutory scheme where this is attributable to *physical* injury also sustained in the accident. This requirement was seen as necessary to avoid stress claims entering "through the back door".

26.   ARCIA 1992 provides that if personal injury by accident is covered by the Act no proceedings can be brought in any court in New Zealand in respect of it.[83] There is some confusion as to whether this has the effect of barring an action at common law for psychiatric illness by those who do not also sustain physical injury. If the action is indeed barred by the Act this means that a common law right has been taken away with nothing put in its place. It has been argued that very clear words should be required before such an interpretation is given by the courts,[84] and the prevailing view in New Zealand, in the absence of a decision by the courts, is that where there is no cover under the scheme the common law right to sue revives.[85]

27.   The lack of case law on common law claims for negligently inflicted psychiatric illness makes it difficult to speculate as to the principles which New Zealand courts would apply if such claims were to be revived. In *Furniss v Fitchett*[86] the Supreme Court decided the question of liability according to foreseeability, without regard to any other policy tests. In that case, the plaintiff consulted the defendant, her physician, and made unfounded allegations to him of violence by her husband. The plaintiff's marriage later broke down. The defendant, under pressure, supplied the plaintiff's husband, who was also a patient, with a letter stating that in his opinion the plaintiff required psychiatric treatment. When the plaintiff was shown the letter some time later she suffered shock, and it was held that she was entitled to recover

---

[81]   *Ibid*, s 3.

[82]   *Ibid*, s 3. "Accident" also includes various forms of burns, radiation exposure, inhalation or ingestion, and chemical absorption. See generally, S Todd, "Duties of care: the New Zealand jurisprudence Part 1: General principles of duty" (1993) 9 PN 2, 6.

[83]   ARCIA 1992, s 14(1).

[84]   R Tobin, "Nervous Shock: The Common Law; Accident Compensation?" [1992] NZLJ 282, 287.

[85]   Correspondence with Ms N White, Senior Legal Research Officer, New Zealand Law Commission, 14 July 1992. See D M Carden, "Accident Compensation and lump sums" [1992] NZLJ 404, 407-408, who also discusses the question whether there is a right to sue where cover under the scheme is inadequate.

[86]   [1958] NZLR 396.

damages against the defendant for negligence. Negligence, causing mental distress, was one of the several causes of action alleged in *Bradley v Wingnut Films Ltd*,[87] but this action was dismissed on the basis that the situation did not fall within any established category giving rise to a duty of care and even if it did that duty would not have been breached on the facts: there was no discussion of the authorities relating to psychiatric illness.

CANADA

28. Canadian law permits recovery for shock-induced psychiatric illness where such injury is foreseeable and is proximately related to the negligent act of the tortfeasor.[88] The plaintiff's psychiatric illness must have been occasioned by "shock" in some sense.[89] At one stage it had appeared, from the decision of the British Columbia Supreme Court in *Rhodes v Canadian National Railway Co*,[90] that the scope of the aftermath doctrine, as applied by Canadian courts, was considerably wider than had previously been believed, but the reversal of that decision by the British Columbia Court of Appeal[91] has reaffirmed its relatively narrow limits.

29. In *Rhodes*, the plaintiff's son was killed in a train crash about which the plaintiff first heard on the radio. She suffered many hours of anxiety before learning that her son was among the victims. Some days later, she travelled to the place where the accident had occurred. She was initially denied access to the site of the accident itself, and when she gained access and asked to see the carriage in which her son died she was shown the wrong carriage. This was followed by other incidents which aggravated her state of mind further. At first instance, Maczko J awarded damages to the plaintiff. In doing so, he claimed support for his view in the reasoning of Deane J in *Jaensch v Coffey*[92] and in the earlier decision of the British Columbia Court of Appeal in *Beecham v Hughes*.[93] He acknowledged that his decision broke new ground, in so far as he could find no case in which damages had been awarded

---

[87] [1993] 1 NZLR 415 (High Ct; Gallen J). The plaintiff owned the right in perpetuity to a burial plot in a cemetery. The defendant film company, with the consent of the cemetery's owners, made a horror film there, and when this came to the attention of the plaintiff he suffered distress. Damages for mental distress were awarded by the Court of Appeal for a solicitor's negligence causing economic loss in *Mouat v Clark Boyce* [1992] 2 NZLR 559: Cooke P, at pp 568-569, distinguished *Alcock v Chief Constable of South Yorkshire Police* [1992] 1 AC 310 as dealing with the different question of whether a duty of care should be owed in respect of psychiatric illness.

[88] See, eg, *Beecham v Hughes* (1988) 52 DLR (4th) 625, in which the British Columbia Court of Appeal adopted the reasoning of Deane J in the Australian case *Jaensch v Coffey* (1984) 155 CLR 549, 606-607, for which see Appendix, paras 8-11 above.

[89] See *Beecham v Hughes* (1988) 52 DLR (4th) 625.

[90] (1989) 49 CCLT 64.

[91] (1990) 75 DLR (4th) 248.

[92] See Appendix, para 8 above.

[93] (1988) 52 DLR (4th) 625.

on the basis of what a plaintiff heard in the absence of firsthand perception, but he thought that *Beecham* had removed this apparently arbitrary limit and had left the door open to recovery in this situation. This reasoning was strongly rejected by the British Columbia Court of Appeal, which held that the plaintiff had insufficient proximity to the accident to enable her to recover. Macfarlane JA disagreed with the conclusion that *Beecham* left open the possibility of recovery in cases where the plaintiff was informed of a loved one's death by a third party without experiencing the shock of the event itself.[94] Taylor JA (with Wood JA concurring) applied the concept of causal proximity discussed in *Jaensch*, but concluded that this concept included elements of physical proximity.[95] Wallace JA appeared to reject the concept of causal proximity, as opposed to a proximity composed of relational, temporal and locational factors.[96]

30. A similarly strict view was taken, and *Rhodes* was followed, in *Strong v Moon*.[97] The plaintiff child sought damages for psychiatric illness sustained as a result of her mother's involvement in a road accident which occurred after her mother had dropped her off at school. The child was told by children who had passed the scene of the accident in a school bus that her mother was seriously injured, but she was subsequently told by the school authorities that her mother was not in fact badly hurt and would recover. However, the child developed long-lasting psychological effects which necessitated treatment. The court held that no duty of care was owed to the plaintiff by the motorist involved in the accident, in that there was no geographical proximity to the shocking event, or any immediacy or directness of impact that would generate a duty of care.[98]

31. In none of these cases were the Canadian courts required to consider the state of the law in relation to the class of claimants entitled to recover damages for psychiatric illness. In *Grzywacz v Vanderheide*,[99] however, the Ontario Court of Justice awarded damages for psychiatric illness to an elderly sister of the deceased, even though the deceased was visiting Canada from Poland, albeit with a view to emigrating there, and so there must have been a degree of separation between the

---

[94] (1990) 75 DLR (4th) 248, 251.

[95] *Ibid*, 295.

[96] *Ibid*, 265.

[97] (1992) 13 CCLT (2d) 296 (BC Sup Ct).

[98] See also *Cormier v Dixon* (1992) 127 NBR (2d) 358 (NB QB), affirmed (1992) 130 NBR (2d) 69 (NB CA) (application for move to strike out claim allowed; the statement of claim did not allege that the plaintiff saw the collision in question or that she was even still present at the scene when it occurred). On the separate question of whether a plaintiff who has received bad news which is untrue and suffered psychiatric illness as a result can recover damages from the person communicating the "news", see *Guay v Sun Publishing Co* [1953] 4 DLR 577 (Sup Ct of Canada). See para 2.48 above.

[99] (30 December 1992, unreported).

plaintiff and the deceased sister. There is an obiter dictum of the British Columbia Supreme Court in *Beaulieu v Sutherland*[100] that, whether the question be viewed as a matter of pure foreseeability or as a matter of policy, the possibility of recovery of damages by persons other than close relatives of the primary victim should be left open.[101] It was suggested in *Beaulieu* that a close friend of the primary victim might in principle be able to recover damages, although on the facts of that case the plaintiff failed for other reasons. In *Bechard v Haliburton Estate*[102] the Ontario Court of Appeal had the opportunity of dealing with this point squarely but it did not take it. In that case the plaintiff was a passenger in a car. The first defendant (who was not known to the plaintiff) had failed to comply with a stop sign on his motorcycle and hit the car in which the plaintiff was sitting. Another car driven by the second defendant, who had been drinking, ran over the first defendant despite the plaintiff's attempt to warn the second defendant, and killed him. The plaintiff recovered damages from the second defendant for psychiatric illness caused, as to 75%, by witnessing the first defendant's death.[103] The court decided the case on the basis that she was in a role similar to that of rescuer. It did not make it clear whether, in cases other than those involving rescuers, the existence of a blood relationship between the plaintiff and the primary victim is required before the plaintiff can recover for psychiatric illness.

32. It appears that a plaintiff cannot recover damages for psychiatric illness arising out of the death or injury caused to the defendant by the defendant's own negligence. In *Cady v Anderson*,[104] an unreported decision of the British Columbia Supreme Court, it was held, *inter alia*, that the plaintiff could not recover damages from her deceased fiancé's estate for psychiatric illness as a result of witnessing the death of her fiancé in a car accident because the deceased was responsible for the accident.

---

[100] (1986) 35 CCLT 237.

[101] *Ibid*, 247-248, *per* Legg J.

[102] (1991) 84 DLR (4th) 668.

[103] It was found that the psychiatric illness was caused, as to the remaining 25%, by the impact of the initial collision with the first defendant. The first defendant's estate was held liable, on appeal, for 25% of the total damage under this head. Although the plaintiff had been receiving treatment for anxiety and depression for some years before the accident, the trial judge had found that this condition did not make her especially vulnerable to the post-traumatic stress disorder which she suffered after the accident. The Ontario Court of Appeal held that, in any case, it was reasonably foreseeable that an average person would have suffered shock-induced psychiatric illness in these circumstances, and therefore the plaintiff was entitled to recover damages for any more extensive illness which she would have suffered as a result of such vulnerability.

[104] 25 November 1992 - File No 14933; 17765. There is a summary of the case in 37 ACWS 3d 46.

THE UNITED STATES

33. American courts have, on the whole, tended to be slower to recognise claims for mental harm[105] than courts in England and other common law jurisdictions. Very importantly, however, in many states there is a lack of rigid distinction between psychiatric illness and mere mental distress, both of which are regarded as compensatable in principle, although a seriousness threshold is adopted.[106]

34. Although the original "impact rule", requiring contemporaneous physical injury, has been abandoned as a limitation on claims for mental distress by the majority of states,[107] many states[108] still follow the "zone of danger" approach prescribed by the Restatement (Second) of Torts.[109] The zone of danger rule, similar to the one laid down in the English case *Dulieu v White*,[110] permits plaintiffs to recover for emotional distress without physical impact if they are placed at risk of physical harm by the conduct in question.[111]

---

[105] See, eg, *Rickey v Chicago Transit Authority* (1983) 457 NE 2d 1 (Illinois). See also *Stadler v Cross* (1980) 295 NW 2d 552 (Minnesota); *Shelton v Russell Pipe and Foundry Co* (1978) 570 SW 2d 861 (Tennessee); *Guilmette v Alexander* (1969) 259 A 2d 12, 14 (Vermont). See R A Chesley, "The Increasingly Disparate Standards of Recovery for Negligently Inflicted Emotional Injuries" (1983) 52 Cincinnati LR 1017, 1031.

[106] See paras 42-43 below.

[107] These are listed in *Gates v Richardson* (1986) 719 P 2d 193, 195 n 1 (Wyoming). The physical impact requirement remains the primary limitation device for mental distress actions in a few jurisdictions, namely Arkansas, District of Columbia, Georgia, Indiana, Kentucky and Oregon: see D B Marlowe, "Negligent Infliction of Mental Distress" (1988) 33 Villanova LR 781, n 59.

[108] Some 20 jurisdictions: see para 5.4 n 5 above.

[109] Section 313 of the Restatement (Second) of Torts (1965) provides:

(1) If the actor unintentionally causes emotional distress to another, he is subject to liability to the other for resulting illness or bodily harm if the actor

(a) should have realised that his conduct involved an unreasonable risk of causing the distress, otherwise than by knowledge of the harm or peril of a third person, and

(b) from facts known to him should have realised that the distress, if it were caused, might result in illness or bodily harm.

(2) The rule stated in Subsection (1) has no application to illness or bodily harm of another which is caused by emotional distress arising solely from harm or peril to a third person, *unless the negligence of the actor has otherwise created an unreasonable risk of bodily harm to the other*. (emphasis added)

[110] [1901] 2 KB 669. See para 2.12 above.

[111] See, for example, *Tebbutt v Virostek* (1985) 483 NE 2d 1142 (New York); *Williams v Baker* (1990) 572 A 2d 1062 (Dist of Columbia); *Asaro v Cardinal Glennon Memorial Hospital* (1990) 799 SW 2d 595 (Missouri); *Hansen v Sea Ray Boats Inc* (1992) 830 P 2d 236 (Utah).

35.   Recognition of the inherent flaws of the zone of danger rule has led some states to adopt a markedly more flexible approach and to permit recovery for distress where the plaintiff witnesses injury to another without being in danger himself or herself.[112] This development was spearheaded by the majority decision of the California Supreme Court in *Dillon v Legg*.[113] The court thought that traditional negligence principles were sufficient to keep liability within reasonable bounds; a duty of care would therefore only be owed to those who were foreseeably exposed, by the defendant's conduct, to the risk of mental distress. In similar fashion to Lord Wilberforce's speech in *McLoughlin v O'Brian*,[114] and to the House of Lords' decision in *Alcock v Chief Constable of South Yorkshire Police*[115] in England, it identified three factors or guidelines to the determination of the defendant's duty in a mental distress case: (1) the plaintiff's physical proximity to the scene of the accident, (2) whether shock resulted from a direct emotional impact upon the plaintiff caused by the sensory and contemporaneous observation of the accident, as contrasted with learning of the accident from others after its occurrence, and (3) the proximity of the relationship between the plaintiff and the victim.[116]

(1) The status of *Dillon*

36.   The American courts showed a mixed reaction to the decision in *Dillon*. Some jurisdictions adopted the *Dillon* criteria.[117] A few have expressed a willingness to do so if an appropriate test case came along.[118] The decision has not, however, received widespread judicial acceptance,[119] and many states refuse altogether to allow a secondary victim to recover for negligent infliction of emotional distress.[120] Some have added other requirements to the three identified in *Dillon*. In *Barnhill v Davis*,[121] for example, the Iowa Supreme Court required in addition that the distress should be serious and that a reasonable person in the position of the secondary victim would believe, and the secondary victim did believe, that the direct victim

---

[112] See L J Rose, "Negligent Infliction of Emotional Distress: Formulating the Psycho-Legal Inquiry" (1984) 18 Suffolk University LR 401, 406.

[113] (1968) 441 P 2d 912. The court in this case discarded the zone of danger requirement and allowed recovery to a mother who had witnessed injury to her child from a position of personal safety.

[114] [1983] 1 AC 410, 416-423. See paras 2.16-2.17 above.

[115] [1992] 1 AC 310.

[116] (1968) 441 P 2d 912, 920.

[117] These are listed by D B Marlowe in "Negligent Infliction of Mental Distress" (1988) 33 Villanova LR 781, 806, n 139.

[118] *Ibid*, 806-807.

[119] See R A Chesley, "The Increasingly Disparate Standards of Recovery for Negligently Inflicted Emotional Injuries" (1983) 52 Cincinnati LR 1017, 1022.

[120] *Ibid*, 1023.

[121] (1981) 300 NW 2d 104.

would be seriously injured or killed.[122] The court also limited the required relationship between victim and plaintiff to spouses or relatives within the second degree of consanguinity or affinity.[123]

37. Of those jurisdictions which adopted the *Dillon* approach, there was disagreement as to the weight to be given to the factors identified by the court in that case and their definition. In California itself, the courts sometimes applied the *Dillon* factors as rigid requirements or doctrinal barriers, as opposed to guidelines, and in particular the requirement that the plaintiff should be at the scene and witness the accident. Thus in *Arauz v Gerhardt*,[124] for example, recovery was denied to a mother who came upon the scene of a motor accident involving her son within five minutes of the accident.[125] On the other hand, in *Ochoa v Superior Court of Santa Clara County* the Supreme Court of California described the strict and mechanical interpretation of the *Dillon* guidelines as giving rise to arbitrary, inconsistent and inequitable results.[126]

38. The flexible approach to the guidelines, at any rate as far as California is concerned, seems to have come to an end with the decision of the Supreme Court of California in *Thing v La Chusa*,[127] in which a mother was out of sight and hearing of the accident which badly injured her son. She was, however, nearby, and she came to

---

[122] *Ibid*, 108.

[123] A small number of states have placed greatest emphasis on the relationship factor in *Dillon*. See, eg, *Portee v Jaffee* (1980) 417 A 2d 521 (New Jersey).

[124] (1977) 68 Cal App 3d 937; 137 Cal Rptr 619.

[125] See also *Parsons v Superior Court for the County of Monterey* (1978) 981 Cal App 3d 506; 146 Cal Rptr 495. In this case the plaintiffs were following their daughters in a car when the defendant driver of the daughters' car crashed. The parents did not see the accident, but arrived on the scene "before the dust had settled". The court held that the plaintiffs did not have a contemporaneous observation of the injury-producing event and therefore dismissed the case. See, further, *Hathaway v Superior Court of Fresno County* (1980) 112 Cal App 3d 728; 169 Cal Rptr 435. The victim in this case was electrocuted on an outdoor cooler; the parents, who were indoors, ran outside to find their son lying in a pool of water, gagging and spitting. The child did not die until later, and the court held that the parents had not contemporaneously observed the event because the child was no longer touching the cooling unit when they arrived. See, too, *Madigan v City of Santa Ana* (1983) 145 Cal App 3d 607; 193 Cal Rptr 593. In *Gates v Richardson* (1986) 719 P 2d 193 (Wyoming) the court stated that "The essence of the tort is the shock caused by the perception of an especially horrendous event...It is more than bad news...It may be the crushed body, the bleeding, the cries of pain, and, in some cases, the dying words": *ibid*, 199. See generally, R N Pearson, "Liability to Bystanders for Negligently Inflicted Emotional Harm - A Comment on the Nature of Arbitrary Rules" (hereafter referred to as "Liability to Bystanders for Negligently Inflicted Emotional Harm") (1982) 4 University of Florida LR 477, 492-495; L J Rose, "Negligent Infliction of Emotional Distress: Formulating the Psycho-Legal Inquiry" (1984) 18 Suffolk University LR 401, 409, n 67 and accompanying text.

[126] (1985) 703 P 2d 1, 17 (Bird CJ). See D B Marlowe, "Negligent Infliction of Emotional Distress" (1988) 33 Villanova LR 781, 814 and accompanying notes.

[127] (1989) 771 P 2d 814.

the site of the accident as soon as she heard about it and saw her son, unconscious and covered in blood. Nevertheless, it was held that she could not recover damages since she had not been at the scene at the time of the accident. The majority of the seven judges heavily criticised the uncertainty which had been created by the cases following *Dillon*, and held that to succeed in recovering damages for emotional distress in third-party situations where the plaintiff had not suffered physical injury, three strict conditions had to be fulfilled: first, that the plaintiff be closely related to the primary victim; secondly, that the plaintiff be present at the scene of the injury-producing event at the time it occurs and be aware that it is causing injury to the primary victim; and thirdly, that, as a result, the plaintiff suffers serious emotional distress beyond that which would be anticipated in a disinterested witness, and which is not an abnormal response to the circumstances.[128] The indications are that the Californian courts are applying these rules strictly.[129]

39. Meanwhile, the courts in other jurisdictions adopted a relaxed approach and interpreted the *Dillon* guidelines quite broadly. Recovery has been permitted, for example, where plaintiffs have arrived at the scene shortly after the accident while the primary victims were still there - at least where the relationship between the two parties was close.[130] Other jurisdictions are yet more liberal and allow recovery, for example, where the plaintiff is "directly involved in the event."[131] *Hearing* the event in question may even be sufficient in some states.[132] In *Paugh v Hanks* the Supreme Court of Ohio emphasised that the *Dillon* factors "were not intended to be fixed guidelines with [sic] which an aggrieved plaintiff-bystander was required to satisfy in order to recover; rather, the factors were to be taken into account by courts in assessing the degree of foreseeability of emotional injury to the plaintiff."[133] However, whilst the court acknowledged the virtue of flexibility in the courts'

---

[128] *Ibid*, 829-830.

[129] See, eg, *Fife v Astenius* (1991) 232 Cal App 3d 1090; 284 Cal Rptr 16.

[130] See *Landreth v Reed* (1978) 570 SW 2d 486 (Texas); *Dziokonski v Babineau* (1978) 380 NE 2d 1295, 1302-1303 (Massachusetts); and *Corso v Merrill* (1979) 406 A 2d 300 (New Hampshire). In *Ferriter v Daniel O'Connell's Sons, Inc* (1980) 413 NE 2d 690 (Massachusetts) the decision allowing the action to proceed was based upon seeing the victim husband and father in hospital some time after the accident which caused his injuries, and in *Campbell v Animal Quarantine Station* (1981) 632 P 2d 1066 (Hawaii), the plaintiffs were awarded damages for emotional distress resulting from the death of their dog in the defendant's possession although the plaintiffs did not witness this. See also D B Marlowe, "Negligent Infliction of Emotional Distress" (1988) 33 Villanova LR 781, 811, nn 165, 169-172 and accompanying text for examples of the disparate treatment given by the courts to the terms used in the *Dillon* guidelines.

[131] *Champion v Gray* (1985) 478 So 2d 17, 20. The Supreme Court of Florida indicated that it would allow recovery where the plaintiff first sees the victim in hospital, as the plaintiff did in *McLoughlin*.

[132] See, eg, *Corso v Merrill* (1979) 406 A 2d 300 (New Hampshire).

[133] (1983) 451 NE 2d 759, 764, approved by the Supreme Court of Nebraska in *James v Lieb* (1985) 375 NW 2d 109.

response, it did modify the *Dillon* requirements so as to require either a marital or intimate familial relationship between the plaintiff and victim, believing that this would serve to limit recovery to those who were most genuinely injured.[134] It remains to be seen how the stricter regime contemplated by *Thing v La Chusa* will affect the other jurisdictions.

40.   Generally, liability in America for emotional injury resulting from apprehension of harm to another has not been extended beyond the situation where a close family member is involved.[135] The recognised categories of relationships which are sufficiently close to enable recovery are usually strictly enforced, so that where a plaintiff's relationship with the primary victim falls outside those categories the plaintiff's claim will usually fail, even if that relationship is analogous to one which does fall within the recognised categories.[136] Recovery has been denied, for example, to an unmarried cohabitant of the injured person.[137]

(2) A general foreseeability analysis

41.   The three proximity factors identified by the California Supreme Court in *Dillon* have, therefore, been given radically differing interpretations by the courts of different states.[138] However, even the most liberal interpretation does not suggest

---

[134] 375 NW 2d 109, 115.

[135] See J D Lee and B A Lindahl, *Modern Tort Law: Liability and Litigation* (Revised ed, 1990) vol 3, para 32.16. Wyoming has defined the necessary relationship through recourse to the state's wrongful death statute: *Gates v Richardson* (1986) 719 P 2d 193. Recovery is limited to spouses, children, parents and siblings. Similarly, Iowa requires that the plaintiff and victim be husband and wife, or related within the second degree of consanguinity: *Barnhill v Davis* (1981) 300 NW 2d 104. Florida requires an "especially close emotional attachment" to the injured party: *Champion v Gray* (1985) 478 So 2d 17; Montana, a close relationship: *Versland v Caron Transport* (1983) 671 P 2d 583, and Arizona requires that the bystander and victim be closely related by consanguinity or otherwise: *Keck v Jackson* (1979) 593 P 2d 668, 670. See D B Marlowe, "Negligent Infliction of Emotional Distress" (1988) 33 Villanova LR 781, 809, n 149 and accompanying text.

[136] But see *Leong v Takasaki* (1974) 520 P 2d 758 (the Supreme Court of Hawaii thought the relationship requirement might be fulfilled even though plaintiff and victim, step-grandson and step-grandmother respectively, had only known each other a few months). See also *Mobaldi v Board of Regents of the University of California* (1976) 55 Cal App 3d 573; 127 Cal Rptr 720 in which the California Court of Appeal reasoned that since emotional attachment rather than legal status determines the closeness of a relationship, it would not require the plaintiff to show blood relationship, marriage or adoption in order to prevail (recovery allowed by primary victim's foster mother. The child was three and a half years old at the date of the accident and had lived with the plaintiff from the time he was 5 months old): *ibid*, at pp 582-583 and 726-727.

[137] *Elden v Sheldon* (1988) 758 P 2d 582; *Drew v Drake* (1980) 110 Cal App 3d 555, 557-58; 168 Cal Rptr 65, 65-66. However, the decision is consistent with the earlier case of *Tong v Jocson* (1977) 76 Cal App 3d 603; 142 Cal Rptr 726 which held that loss of consortium actions cannot be maintained with respect to an engaged couple living together at the time of the accident. See also *Coon v Joseph* (1987) 192 Cal App 3d 1269; 237 Cal Rptr 873, in which a male plaintiff failed to recover as a witness to the assault of an "intimate male friend" because such a relationship failed to satisfy the "close relationship" requirement of *Dillon*.

[138] B S Markesinis, *The German Law of Torts* (3rd ed 1994) pp 126-128.

that foreseeability is the only test for recovery.[139] A few courts, however, have extended liability beyond the quite rigid *Dillon* guidelines to a general foreseeability analysis.[140] In *Hunsley v Giard*,[141] for example, the Supreme Court of Washington reasoned that liability would be kept within reasonable bounds by limiting the defendant's duty to foreseeable plaintiffs and requiring objective symptomatology of emotional suffering,[142] and in *Bass v Nooney Co* the Supreme Court of Missouri set out a two-prong test permitting recovery where (1) the defendant should have realised that his conduct created an unreasonable risk of creating emotional distress and (2) the emotional distress was medically diagnosable and of sufficient severity to be medically significant.[143]

(3) The physical manifestation and severity tests

42.　In some jurisdictions, it is necessary to establish that the emotional distress suffered by the plaintiff has manifested itself in physical symptoms.[144] Application of this test has also often, but not invariably, coincided with the zone of danger test. The court in *Dillon* did not have to decide whether physical symptoms were present because, on the facts, they clearly were. In *Molien v Kaiser Foundation Hospitals*[145] however, the Supreme Court of California dispensed with the requirement, and proof of "serious mental distress" will now suffice.[146] Other jurisdictions which follow the *Dillon* analysis are split on whether there is a need for such a physical manifestation

---

[139] See R N Pearson, "Negligently Inflicted Emotional Harm" (1982) 4 University of Florida LR 477, 497-499. Pearson suggests that what may have emerged from the post-*Dillon* line of cases is an open-ended "take-into-account-all-the-circumstances" rule under which a court might balance the strength of one factor in the plaintiff's case with a weakness in another. Alternatively, what has evolved may be even more vague such that it is more of an "approach" than a rule.

[140] D B Marlowe, "Negligent Infliction of Mental Distress" (1988) 33 Villanova LR 781, 810, 813-817, and n 160.

[141] (1976) 553 P 2d 1096 (Washington).

[142] *Ibid*, 1103. See also *Rodrigues v State* (1970) 472 P 2d 509, 520 (Hawaii); *Sinn v Burd* (1979) 404 A 2d 672, 683 (Pennsylvania); *Culbert v Sampson's Supermarkets Inc* (1982) 444 A 2d 433, 437 (Maine); *Croft v Wicker* (1987) 737 P 2d 789 (Alaska). See generally N Quay-Smith, "The Negligent Infliction of Emotional Distress" (1986) 19 Indiana LR 809, 814-817.

[143] (1983) 646 SW 765, 772-773.

[144] See, eg, *Champion v Gray* (1985) 478 So 2d 17 (Florida); *Payton v Abbott Labs* (1982) 437 NE 2d 171 (Massachusetts); *Corso v Merrill* (1979) 406 A 2d 300 (New Hampshire); *Ramirez v Armstrong* (1983) 673 P 2d 822 (New Mexico); *Curtis v State Department for Children and Their Families* (1987) 522 A 2d 203 (Rhode Island).

[145] (1980) 616 P 2d 813.

[146] At least where the plaintiff is a "direct victim" of the defendant's negligence (in *Molien*, the defendant-doctor negligently misdiagnosed the plaintiff's wife as having a venereal disease and advised her to urge her husband to have treatment. The stress and suspicion of sexual infidelity caused the marriage to dissolve. The court held that the plaintiff-husband was a direct victim of the defendant's negligence).

of distress.[147]

43.   Where the physical manifestation test is not applied, claims for emotional distress are generally subject to a requirement that the distress should be of a particular degree of severity.[148] Medical testimony is not required to prove severity. Lay testimony might show the effects of emotional distress by recounting the plaintiff's withdrawal from society or deteriorating physical appearance, or a family's testimony might illustrate the relationship the plaintiff had with the victim and the distress caused by the loss.[149]

---

[147] See D B Marlowe, "Negligent Infliction of Mental Distress" (1988) 33 Villanova LR 781, 808 and accompanying notes.

[148] *Molien v Kaiser Foundation Hospitals* (1980) 616 P 2d 813 (California); *Leong v Takasaki* (1974) 520 P 2d 758 (Hawaii); *Rodrigues v State* (1970) 472 P 2d 509 (Hawaii); *Culbert v Sampson's Supermarkets Inc* (1982) 444 A 2d 433, 437 (Maine); *Ferriter v Daniel O'Connell's Sons, Inc* (1980) 413 NE 2d 690 (Massachusetts); *Bass v Nooney Co* (1982) 646 SW 2d 765, 772-773 (Missouri); *Portee v Jaffee* (1980) 417 A 2d 521 (New Jersey); *Paugh v Hanks* (1983) 451 NE 2d 759, 765 (Ohio); *Schultz v Barberton Glass Co* (1983) 447 NE 2d 109, 112-113 (Ohio). Attempts to describe the necessary seriousness of injury have included the following: "emotional distress...as severe and debilitating as physical harm" (*Molien v Kaiser Foundation Hospitals* (1980) 616 P 2d 813, 814, California) while V Nolan and E Ursin state that the seriousness criterion "refers to severe and debilitating emotional injury with its attendant painful mental suffering and anguish - injury of grave intensity and duration": "Negligent Infliction of Emotional Distress: Coherence Emerging from Chaos" (1982) 33 Hastings LJ 583, 615. Institutionalisation or hospitalisation might be an indication of the severity of the illness (*Archibold v Braverman* (1969) 275 Cal App 2d 253; 79 Cal Rptr 723, California), as might being rendered bedridden (*Mobaldi v Board of Regents of University of California* (1976) 55 Cal App 3d 573; 127 Cal Rptr 720, California) or incapable of performing ordinary household duties, together with loss of weight combined with nervousness or irritability (*Daley v LaCroix* (1970) 179 NW 2d 390, Michigan) and withdrawal from normal forms of socialisation (*Toms v McConnell* (1973) 207 NW 2d 140, Michigan). In articulating standards for recovery, the courts of those States which employ a seriousness criterion have identified common physiological reactions illustrative of the types of disorders often associated with severe emotional distress. However, proof that emotional injury is severe and debilitating does not necessitate the introduction of expert medical testimony on this point. Other proposed solutions to the problem of fraudulent and trivial claims have included the suggestion that damages should be limited to pecuniary or economic out-of-pocket losses such as wages and medical expenses.

[149] See, eg, *Vance v Vance* (1979) 408 A 2d 728, 734-735 (Maryland). The plaintiff's condition need not amount to a recognisable psychiatric illness, although the plaintiff may show the requisite level of severity by establishing, by way of expert medical testimony, the "medically significant nature" of his or her condition (*Bass v Nooney Co* (1986) 646 SW 2d 765) or that it is "medically diagnosable" (*ibid*; *Davis v Shelton* (1986) 710 SW 2d 8): *Molien v Kaiser Foundation Hospitals* (1980) 616 P 2d 813, 821. See V Nolan and E Ursin, "Negligent Infliction of Emotional Distress: Coherence Emerging from Chaos" (1982) 33 Hastings LJ 583, 615, 618-619; and L J Rose, "Negligent Infliction of Emotional Distress: Formulating the Psycho-Legal Inquiry" (1984) 18 Suffolk University LR 401, 425-427. However, the American courts have reiterated that the best indication of a claim's genuineness is the jurors' reference to their own experience as opposed to medical testimony: see *Molien v Kaiser Foundation Hospitals* (1980) 616 P 2d 813, 821. However, it may be that it is easier to formulate a test than to apply it: B S Markesinis, *The German Law of Torts* (3rd ed 1994) p 120.

FRANCE

44.   The French Civil Code contains a general principle of liability for fault. Article 1382 provides that a person who causes damage to another through fault is liable to compensate that other.[150] The case law clearly establishes that this covers both economic injury (*dommage matériel*) and injury which is non-economic in nature (*dommage moral*);[151] and further that *dommage moral* extends to include not only a psychiatric illness but also mere mental distress, such as grief and anxiety, even where this is not consequential on any bodily injury. Claims brought by someone who is not the immediate victim of the defendant's fault for *dommage par ricochet*, for example by the grieving parents of a child killed by the defendant's negligence, form a sub-category of *dommages moraux*.[152] Thus, damages may be recovered for mere emotional distress suffered on the death or injury of another.[153] However, this wide principle of liability is tempered by the causation rules which the courts apply. Although the Code has no provision requiring direct causation in tort cases, the French courts have extended the requirement in contract cases set by Article 1151 to tort cases also, with the effect that the injury must be both "direct" and "certain".[154]

45.   Given the generality of Article 1382, it is hard to ascertain the precise limits of liability for negligence in French law,[155] and claims brought by those who are not the immediate victim of the defendant's fault have given rise to some difficulty in the past.[156] The major difficulty has concerned the size of the class entitled to seek compensation under Article 1382, which at one time appeared to be confined to

---

[150] Article 1383 provides that a person is responsible not only for damage caused by intentional actions, but also for that caused by negligence or carelessness.

[151] G Ripert, *La Règle morale dans les obligations civiles* (1949) para 181; B Starck, *Droit civil, obligations* (2nd ed 1985) vol 1, paras 110-122; F H Lawson, A E Anton & L Neville Brown, *Amos & Walton's Introduction to French Law* (3rd ed 1967) pp 209-210.

[152] See generally B Starck, *Droit civil, obligations* (2nd ed 1985) vol 1, paras 123, 146-159.

[153] In English law, claims by secondary victims for mental injury in respect of the negligently caused injury or death of another can only take the form of a claim for psychiatric injury within the parameters of *Alcock* [1992] 1 AC 310 or for bereavement damages under s 1A(1) of the Fatal Accidents Act 1976, as inserted by s 3 of the Administration of Justice Act 1982. We will be examining bereavement damages in a forthcoming consultation paper.

[154] F H Lawson, A E Anton & L Neville Brown, *Amos & Walton's Introduction to French Law* (3rd ed 1967) p 213; B Starck, *Droit civil, obligations* (2nd ed 1985) vol 1, para 836.

[155] F H Lawson, *Negligence in the Civil Law* (1950) p 31; M G Bridge, "Contractual Damages for Intangible Loss: A Comparative Analysis" (1984) 62 Can BR 323, 332, n 32, 335-336. In 1962, the Cour de Cassation awarded damages to an owner and a trainer for their distress on the death of a racehorse. Bridge, *ibid* at 336, remarks that the decision "is widely regarded as having taken '*dommage moral*' liability too far.... Its legacy is the impossibility thus created of knowing where liability stops."

[156] M G Bridge, *ibid*, 337.

close relations. Although this restriction no longer operates,[157] it seems that the courts will apply causation rules flexibly so as to exclude extravagant claims. The more remote the relationship between the immediate victim and the victim *par ricochet*, the less likely it is that the latter will be able to establish that his or her injury is "direct" and "certain".[158] Where the immediate victim dies as a result of his or her injuries, it seems that anyone who suffers mental injury may recover damages,[159] provided he or she is able to show that the injury amounts to a real and sufficiently profound sadness ("*douleur vraiment profonde*").[160] In practice, courts tend to presume its existence in the case of certain near relatives, especially the deceased's parents, husband, wife and children.[161] Where the immediate victim is merely injured, a more limited class (which includes relatives and fiancé(e)s) may recover.[162] However, in both instances the victim *par ricochet* may recover damages for mental distress regardless of whether he or she witnessed the accident to the immediate victim and regardless of whether the mental distress is shock-induced. French law therefore goes much further than English law in recognising, in principle at least, widespread liability for negligently caused mental injury standing alone, subject only to the limiting effect of flexible notions of fault and causation.

GERMANY[163]

46. Negligently inflicted psychiatric illness has been held by the German courts to comprise injury to health within Article 823(1) of the German Civil Code. It must, however, entail a medically recognisable psychiatric illness; mere fright, anguish, distress or grief will not suffice.[164] This principle was affirmed in an appeal decided

---

[157] F H Lawson, A E Anton & L Neville Brown, *Amos & Walton's Introduction to French Law* (3rd ed 1967) p 210, observe that the potential class of persons who may suffer grief as a result of death is virtually limitless and that, although it could be delimited on the basis of relationship, there is no text to justify such a restriction in France.

[158] H & L Mazeaud & A Tunc, *Traité théorique et pratique de la responsabilité civile délictuelle et contractuelle* (6th ed 1965) vol 1, para 324-2 (damage is increasingly difficult to establish with the requisite degree of probity as the relationship with the deceased becomes more remote); M G Bridge, "Contractual Damages for Intangible Loss: A Comparative Analysis" (1984) 62 Can BR 323, 338.

[159] For instance, damages were recovered by a mistress in a decision of the Cour de Cassation in 1970. See N J Mullany & P R Handford, *Tort Liability for Psychiatric Damage* (1993) p 102, n 75.

[160] H & L Mazeaud & A Tunc, *Traité théorique et pratique de la resposibilité civile délictuelle et contractuelle* (6th ed 1965) vol 1, paras 324-2 and 325-2; F H Lawson, A E Anton & L Neville Brown, *Amos & Walton's Introduction to French Law* (3rd ed 1967) p 210.

[161] F H Lawson, A E Anton & L Neville Brown, *ibid*.

[162] See N J Mullany & P R Handford, *Tort Liability for Psychiatric Damage* (1993) p 102.

[163] We gratefully acknowledge that we have relied heavily in this summary on Professor B S Markesinis's *The German Law of Torts* (3rd ed 1994).

[164] (1971) 56 BGHZ 163.

by the *Bundesgerichtshof*[165] in 1989.[166] The plaintiff's 22-year-old son was killed in a road accident involving the defendant. Because of their state of mind the plaintiff and her husband cancelled their holiday, which had been due to start on the day after the funeral. Their action against the defendant included a claim for the cost of the foregone holiday. This was refused on appeal on the basis that, *inter alia*, although they had undoubtedly suffered grief and psychological pressure, the symptoms suffered did not display an obvious pathology and accordingly did not constitute an injury to health within the meaning of Article 823(1).

47. German law adopts a more liberal view than English law in that compensation is recoverable where a relative's psychiatric illness is attributable to receipt of the news of the accident.[167] In its judgment of 21 September 1931 the *Reichsgericht*[168] decided that in cases of psychiatric illness caused by negligence two questions must be decided, namely, whether the causal nexus could be regarded as adequate and, if so, whether injury of this type could be foreseen.[169] The case in question involved a mother who had a nervous breakdown upon receiving the news of the death of her seven-year-old son in a road accident. The court found that it was normally to be expected that a mother would suffer great emotional distress by reason of the death of her child in an accident, and that it was entirely foreseeable if this resulted in turn in a nervous breakdown. Four decades later, in 1971, the *Bundesgerichtshof* endorsed the earlier views of the courts that recovery should not be confined to eye-witness relatives but should also be allowed where the injurious effect was distant.[170]

---

[165] Germany's Federal (Supreme) Court, established in 1950 and dealing with civil and criminal matters.

[166] [1989] NJW 2317. See B S Markesinis, *The German Law of Torts* (3rd ed 1994) pp 114-118.

[167] (1929) 133 RGZ 270; (1971) 56 BGHZ 163; (1985) 93 BGHZ 351. See B S Markesinis, *The German Law of Torts* (3rd ed 1994) pp 95-130.

[168] The first supreme court for the whole of Germany, established in 1879 and the pre-cursor to the modern *Bundesgerichtshof* (see para 46 n 165 above).

[169] (1931) 133 RGZ 270. The courts in England have recourse to the notion of the duty of care to deal with the crucial issues in psychiatric illness cases, but German law, in common with other civil law systems, uses normative concepts of causation. Therefore, where the line should eventually be drawn in cases of psychiatric illness is treated as a question of legal cause, although German writers increasingly recognise that the problem is not one of causation but one of policy: B S Markesinis, *The German Law of Torts* (3rd ed 1994) p 39.

[170] (1971) 56 BGHZ 163. In the case in question the plaintiff claimed damages for the injury to her health which she suffered upon hearing of the death of her husband in a traffic accident. See also (1985) 93 BGHZ 351, in which the plaintiff, who was *en ventre sa mère* when her mother was told of her husband's serious injuries in a traffic accident, obtained a declaratory judgment that she was entitled to damages for the physical injuries she suffered at birth because the process of birth was affected by the mother's psychological reaction to the news.

48. The court made the further observation that if the husband's death had been solely attributable to his failure to take care of himself, the plaintiff would have had no claim whatever for compensation for the consequent injury to herself, for to impose a legal duty on a person to look after his own life or limb simply in order to save his dependants from the likely psychiatric effects on them if he is killed or maimed, would be to restrict undesirably his self-determination. The observation was made in the context of the court's view that the contributory negligence of the primary victim would operate to reduce the damages of the secondary victim for psychiatric illness. If contributory negligence were not taken into account, the bar to an action against the primary victim himself would otherwise produce injustice in a situation where the primary victim was much more to blame for his own death than the tortfeasor. "It follows that unless our present view [on the contributory negligence of the primary victim] is adopted, the tortfeasor would owe the shocked widow a full indemnity for her lost earnings even if the husband was so much more to blame for his own death than the tortfeasor that in a suit by the husband the tortfeasor would be wholly exonerated....This would be quite unacceptable."[171]

---

[171] This is from the translation of the case by Tony Weir, reproduced in B S Markesinis, *The German Law of Torts* (3rd ed 1994) p 113.